Praise for *The Anatomy of Addiction*

"A lucid examination of addiction and treatment from a neurobiological perspective . . . with particularly engrossing chapters dispelling the ten biggest myths of addiction."

—*Kirkus Reviews*

"In *The Anatomy of Addiction*, Dr. Mohammad's look at the current addiction treatment climate is direct, unflinching, and an absolute must-read for everyone touched by addiction. The man is a true pioneer in the field of addiction and one of the few addiction experts to accurately and effectively balance science, medicine, and behavioral health. If you want a new perspective on the world of addiction, read this book."

—Darren Kavinoky, co-creator and host of *Deadly Sins* on Investigation Discovery; founding attorney of 1.800.NoCuffs; Certified Intervention Professional

"When I first met Dr. Mohammad, addiction had left me broken and destitute on every level. While I had spent time with countless, self-proclaimed addiction experts, Dr. Mohammad saved and changed my life in a matter of minutes. He was the only treatment professional to let me know that with the help of science, the truth about addiction, and a balanced treatment approach, I could have my life and family back. That was thirteen years ago and I've never looked back. What Dr. Mohammad shared with me that day is included in his book *The Anatomy of Addiction*; we are not powerless over addiction and this book tells you exactly why."

—JW, a patient of Dr. Akikur Mohammad

"This is strong medicine with no spoonful of sugar; for many, it [may be] a bitter pill to swallow. But the book is not meant to inform; it is meant to transform."

—Dr. Walter Ling, professor of psychiatry and director of Integrated Substance Abuse Programs (ISAP) at UCLA

"Dr. Akikur Mohammad is passionate about the issue of addiction, what it is and what it is not, and how it should and shouldn't be treated. Written for the layperson, this book is a helpful resource for readers struggling with addiction, and their families and friends, as well as anyone who is interested in the global problem of addiction."

—George Simpson, MD, professor of psychiatry and the behavioral sciences at Keck School of Medicine at University of Southern Califorinia and former chairman of the department of psychiatry at Keck School of Medicine at University of Southern California

The
Anatomy
of Addiction

What Science and Research
Tell Us About the True Causes,
Best Preventive Techniques,
and Most Successful Treatments

Akikur Mohammad, MD

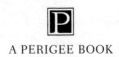

A PERIGEE BOOK

PERIGEE
An imprint of Penguin Random House LLC
375 Hudson Street, New York, New York 10014

Library of Congress Cataloging-in-Publication Data

Names: Mohammad, Akikur, author.
Title: The anatomy of addiction : what science and research tell us about the
true causes, best preventive techniques, and most successful treatments /
Akikur Mohammad, MD.
Description: First edition. | New York City : Perigee, 2016. | Includes
bibliographical references and index.
Identifiers: LCCN 2015041635 | ISBN 978-1-101-98183-2
Subjects: LCSH: Substance abuse—Etiology. | Compulsive behavior—Etiology. |
Substance abuse—Treatment. | BISAC: SELF-HELP / Substance Abuse &
Addictions / General. | PSYCHOLOGY / Psychopathology / Addiction.
Classification: LCC RC564 .M634 2016 | DDC 362.29—dc23

First edition: February 2016

PRINTED IN THE UNITED STATES OF AMERICA

1   3   5   7   9   10   8   6   4   2

Text design by Eve L. Kirch

This book is dedicated to my mother, who inspired me in every way; to my very supportive sister; and to my loving family—my wife, Irina, and our daughters, Anastasia and Sasha.

Contents

viii   Contents

INTRODUCTION

The Invisible Epidemic That's Killing Us

L ast year, the treatment of alcoholism and drug addiction gener-
ated a staggering $34 billion in revenues. Rehab clinics dot the
country and can be found in virtually every city and town in
America. At 14,000 and counting, there are more addiction treatment centers in the United States than there are Starbucks stores.

Yet, the treatment of alcohol and drug addiction is failing
miserably. According to the National Survey on Drug Use and
Health (NSDUH), an estimated 20 million Americans, or about 8
percent of the population, aged twelve or older used an illegal
drug in the past thirty days. In addition, the nonmedical use or
abuse of prescription drugs—including painkillers, sedatives, and
stimulants—is growing, with an estimated 48 million people, or
about 20 percent of the U.S. population, aged twelve and older
using prescription drugs for nonmedical reasons.

To look at it another way, 88,000 deaths were attributable

last year to excessive alcohol use alone in the United States. This makes excessive alcohol use the third leading lifestyle-related cause of death for the nation (it surpassed car accidents in 2009 and never looked back). Excessive alcohol use is responsible for 2.5 million years of potential life lost (YPLL) annually, or an average of about 30 YPLL for each death. In 2006, there were more than 1.2 million emergency room visits and 2.7 million physician office visits due to excessive drinking. The economic cost of excessive alcohol consumption in 2012 was estimated at $275 billion.

The problem of addiction is seemingly everywhere, but the disease of addiction still isn't recognized. If addiction were acknowledged by society—its care providers, the policy makers, the courts and judiciary systems, and most of all, the public—as the chronic disease that it clearly is, it would be quickly brought under control.

In a landmark study of addiction in the United States published by National Center on Addiction and Substance Abuse at Columbia University, the authors found that "addiction is this nation's largest preventable and mostly health problem." They went on to say that the failure to treat addiction with scientifically sound, medically proven methods results in an "enormous array of health and social problems, including accidents, homicides, suicides, child neglect, incarceration and sexual assault."

Admittedly, the figures are so overwhelming that we in the public become desensitized to their effect, until a loved one, friend, or associate succumbs to drug or alcohol abuse. Periodically, when a high-profile figure like Philip Seymour Hoffman dies of an overdose, the country is jolted back to the reality of the dire situation, and the need for changes to addiction treatment are discussed, and then forgotten again until the next celebrity overdose.

But it doesn't have to be so. In the last decade, and, particularly in the last few years, advances have been made in the science of addiction medicine that make the disease both treatable and preventable.

As a board-certified psychiatrist with an additional certification in addiction medicine, I have been on the front line of using these advanced techniques, first, during my work in the emergency room (ER) department of Los Angeles County General Hospital, and now for the last several years at the addiction treatment center I founded in Malibu, California. Yet, I am the first to admit that evidence-based addiction treatment remains largely unknown to the public at large.

Why, then, is there such a disconnect between the problem and the solution? In this book, *The Anatomy of Addiction*, I explain how an entrenched rehab industry has grown scandalously rich by bilking some of the most vulnerable in our society for billions of dollars each year and how it also has no intention of voluntarily changing its way.

Shockingly, an estimated 90 percent of all rehab clinics do not use any evidence-based medicine in their treatment programs. In fact, only six states in the country require any type of education for addiction treatment personnel, often self-styled as "addiction counselors." Instead of offering the kind of proven addiction medicine that has been endorsed by the American Medical Association and National Institutes of Health, these often unscrupulous and always ignorant clinics base their treatment protocols exclusively on 1930s-era concepts of the support talk group concept and enforced abstinence.

Despite decades of scientific research that have proven beyond any reasonable doubt that addiction is a brain disease, the rehab industry continues to treat addiction as a moral failing and lack of willpower. It is abetted in this falsehood by an entrenched establishment that continues to preach its 12-step dogma, despite the facts to the contrary; by policy makers and judiciary, who view the disease as the target for criminalization rather than treatment; by a medical community still largely ignorant of the disease of addiction and its proper treatment; and finally, by a public that is simultaneously supportive and scornful of addicts but mostly just confused by the whole issue.

Here are the simple, scientifically proven facts about alcohol and drug addiction:

1. Addiction is a chronic brain disease, characterized by compulsive craving for alcohol or drugs, that requires medical intervention and management over a lifetime by trained and certified professionals (just like every other chronic disease).
2. Yes, it's a chronic disease of the brain like bipolar disorder, and thus its treatment requires more than counseling and group talk therapy (no matter how good the intentions might be).
3. In fact, alcohol and drug addiction requires first and foremost, pharmacological therapy in addition to counseling and lifestyle modification.

4. As a chronic recurring illness, addiction often requires continued treatment to anticipate relapses and diminish their intensity.

5. While relapses are to be expected, addiction is a treatable condition, and people with an alcohol or drug addiction can recover and lead fulfilling lives.

These guiding principles are at the heart of this book. As you will see, I explain in layman's terms what constitutes effective, evidence-based addiction medicine and how to find it. Just as important, I detail how to avoid so-called rehab clinics that are, at best, useless and a waste of money and, at worst, dangerous and even life-threatening.

The information in this book destroys the myths that, unfortunately, continue to guide addiction treatment in this country, including

- Addiction can be cured by abstinence and willpower.
- Addiction cannot be prevented, and addicts are doomed to life of despair.
- The best form of treatment is advice from former addicts talking about how they kicked their habits.

False, false, and false. Indeed, as a physician, clinician, and professor of medicine, I know of no other medical condition of the brain—be it Alzheimer's disease, Parkinson's disease, or any other—that has amateurs diagnosing and treating it. This simple truth has been proven irrefutable by many scientifically conducted studies: Addiction is a preventable, treatable disease.

In this book you'll find actionable, *scientific* information for addicts and their families. This is the same information that I teach to the students at the Keck School of Medicine of the University of Southern California in Los Angeles. My classes have been considered so essential that regardless of their intended specialties, all med students there are required to take them.

Now, for the first time, I am sharing this information with the public. My goal is nothing less than to once and for all end those who keep addicts and the medical treatment of their disease in the shadows of ignorance, fear, and stigma.

If there is one message you'll take away from this book, it's this: America does not have an addiction problem. It has an addiction *treatment* problem.

The Anatomy of Addiction

Chapter 1

Addiction Is Preventable.
Addiction Is Treatable.

Several years ago, I was a speaker at a conference about addiction medicine during which I called for change in how we think of addicts. If we accept the irrefutable science that drug addiction is a disease, then it follows that we must stop criminalizing addicts' behaviors. Imagine if we criminalized the behavior of other sufferers of leading chronic diseases? Our jails would be filled with people diagnosed with cancer, heart disease, diabetes, and asthma.

After my talk, a gentleman approached me and introduced himself as an agent with the federal Drug Enforcement Agency (DEA). He recounted the story of one of his arrests that continued to haunt him. A heroin pusher had plea-bargained his charge of possession by agreeing to finger accomplices. He identified a couple and, sure enough, a search warrant of their home turned up a couple dozen packages of heroin.

So what was the problem? Their arrest removed dangerous criminals from the streets of Los Angeles, right? In reality, the couple was anything but the stereotype of most people's idea of "heroin addicts." According to the detective, you would have never guessed by looking at the perpetrators that they were abusing drugs. They appeared to be and, in fact, were a middle-class couple living in a nice three-bedroom middle-class home, both holding steady jobs, and neither having been previously arrested for a violent crime.

They were also parents to two young children—a four-year-old girl and seven-year-old boy.

After the man's arrest and conviction (he took the blame), he went to jail, essentially, forever. The woman, depressed and no longer able to get her regular opiate fix, committed suicide. Their kids ended up in foster care.

Even after many years, clearly the detective remained distraught at the havoc his by-the-book arrest had caused to this family. "If I could do it over again, I'd make sure this time that I never found any heroin," he said with conviction. Welcome to the often heart-breaking world of addiction in America.

The Truth About Addiction

In another more just and humane world, the couple at the center of this real-life tragedy would have been diagnosed as having the chronic disease of addiction and provided medical help to end their substance abuse. After a successful evidence-based treatment program, they would have returned to normal, productive lives but without the crutch of substance abuse and the constant fear and stress of being arrested.

Indeed, decades of basic laboratory science have revealed that addiction is a bona fide medical problem involving profound brain alterations. Alcohol, opiates, cocaine, and other substances increase levels of the chemical dopamine in the reward pathway of the brain. With the advent of MRI technology in the late 1970s, we could actually see with our own eyes how addiction depleted baseline dopamine levels, with the net result being a less pleasurable high, requiring ever-larger doses.

Scientifically controlled research studies have revealed that even when people are weaned from a drug, their brains don't return to normal. So such people remain vulnerable to the drug's draw and suffer mood swings and profound urges to use again.

Such findings have been published in science journals at a prodigious rate since the early 2000s, adding weight to the position taken by National Institute on Drug Abuse chief Nora Volkow that "addiction is a chronic disorder that will require multiple rounds of therapy to reduce the risk of relapse and to lengthen drug-free intervals."

In the mid-1990s, a coalition of doctors, scientists, and leading government organizations, including the American Medical Association and the American Psychiatric Association, began pushing for broad recognition of addiction as a disease and advocating more medical approaches to therapy. Gil Kerlikowske, former director of the Office of National Drug Control Policy and President Barack Obama's former top adviser on drug policy, lent clarity to the effort by declaring that addiction "is not a moral failing on the part of the individual. It's a chronic disease of the brain that can be treated."

Despite all the progress in understanding addiction and how to treat it with evidence-based medicine, consider these sobering facts from an in-depth report released by Columbia University in 2013:

- About 21 million Americans have a substance abuse disorder for which they need, but are not receiving, evidence-based addiction treatment.
- Deaths from drug overdoses now exceed traffic fatalities.
- About 55 percent of all prisoners in federal prisons are there for drug-related offenses.
- Nine out of ten people addicted to drugs other than nicotine receive no treatment.
- Most of those who do get treatment are put through unproven programs run by people without medical training.

The Strange History of Addiction in the United States

What accounts for the discrepancy between the availability of modern-day treatment of addiction and its meager use? There are several interrelated reasons, but all have to do with the shame and ignorance surrounding addiction.

First and foremost, public opinion about addiction has not yet caught up with the science. Addicts are still stigmatized by society as moral failures who could cure themselves if they just tried hard enough or, in a variation on this theme, addicts are born losers and there's nothing that can help them.

Let's take the last point first. Judy Garland, Robert Downey Jr., Oprah Winfrey, Bob Dylan, David Bowie, Ray Charles, Keith Urban, Brian Wilson, William F. Buckley Jr., Elizabeth Taylor, James Baldwin, and even Benjamin Franklin were all alcohol and drug addicts. Clearly, these talented and financially successful people were not losers in any conventional sense.

As for the stigma of being an addict, there's no doubt that it's still a powerful force that stops most people from admitting they have an addiction problem. We only have to look at the very high profile and tragic death of actor Philip Seymour Hoffman to confirm this. Here was a celebrated and admired artist, at the top of his career, who nevertheless refused to seek the kind of professional help he needed because of the stigma surrounding a relapse after more than twenty years of sobriety. Instead, he tried curing himself by attending AA meetings. Ten weeks after he relapsed, he was found dead in his apartment with a needle stuck in his arm and seventy-five packages of heroin strewn about.

These public attitudes toward addicts are in part created by America's unique Puritanical history, which underpins our nation's belief system on a wide range of social issues. Americans also tend to think that people who behave badly while drinking or drugging are bona fide addicts. In addition, the vestiges of the late-twentieth-century federal policy known as the "war on drugs" have indelibly etched into the public mind the idea that most drug and alcohol abusers exhibit criminal behavior (when, in fact, only a small minority do).

What history tells us about addiction in America is almost the stuff of fiction. In 1914, the federal government made the fateful decision to criminalize drugs in the United States with the passage of the Harrison Act, designed to limit the distribution of opiate narcotics and to appease the great temperance movement that was sweeping the nation at the time. In 1919, the passage of the Eighteenth Amendment prohibited the sale of alcohol, and by the mid-1920s, the sale and distribution of cannabis were also regulated by federal statue, with criminal penalties attached for those who violated the new rules.

That will be the last time alcohol, narcotics, and cannabis will all be on roughly equal footing in the eyes of the law because, by wildly popular demand, the ban on alcohol became the first and only amendment to the U.S. Constitution that was ever repealed. Alcohol again became readily available, and even glamorized as a lifestyle choice. Meanwhile, marijuana, which was further criminalized, and narcotic opioids diverged onto parallel pathways and were perceived as dangerous, illicit street drugs, along with prescribed painkillers that were considered "safe when used properly." Note though that cannabis is seeing a reversal and has been legalized in some states.

From a medical viewpoint, that made no sense. Alcohol then, and now, by far continues to be the most dangerous drug in terms of the loss of human life and property—more than all other drugs combined. Six people die each day from alcohol poisoning; no one has ever died from a marijuana overdose. And while the country is currently in the midst of a heroin epidemic, it's reflective of the Alice-in-Wonderland world of drug criminalization in the United States that the reason for its resurgence is because the legal version of opiates—prescription painkillers like OxyContin, Percocet, and Demerol—became too scarce on the black market as a result of new federal regulations. Pill addicts turned to heroin, because it became cheaper than prescription painkillers.

If you're looking for any rhyme or reason to how drugs (and alcohol) have been regulated in the United States, you won't find it in history. To add but one more chapter in the surreal saga, the Narcotics Addict Rehabilitation Act of 1966, in a refreshing burst of enlightened thinking, gave judges the discretion to divert a defendant into treatment rather than jail. It was a chink in the armor of the war on drugs begun in 1914.

What the drafters of this act didn't anticipate were the unintended consequences. Suddenly, local communities were encouraged, even expected, to open their own treatment facilities. Local officials, who had virtually no experience in dealing with addicts other than putting them in jail, turned to the only group they knew in the field, Alcoholics Anonymous (AA). But here was the conundrum: co-founder Bill Wilson intended AA to be voluntary. The new law demanded that treatment be regimented with defined time frames and discipline, just like a jail. The rehab industry took off like gangbusters and never looked back.

The Science of Addiction

Here's what science tell us: Addiction is not synonymous with recreational or social use of mood-altering agents, including alcohol. On one level, we all know this intuitively. After all, not everyone who takes a prescription pill, smokes a joint, swigs a cocktail, or even shoots heroin will become an addict. Once we clear up this misunderstanding, then we can begin to realize that addiction is a true medical illness and understand why it is classified as a disease by every medical organization in the world, including the World Health Organization (WHO). Obviously, if addiction were not a medical condition meeting the clear definition of *disease*, my board-certified area of specialization—addiction medicine—wouldn't exist.

Much of the disconnect between addiction and treatment is rooted in the recovery movement's history. Addicts, shunned by society and the medical establishment alike, received their help from those outside of it, a trend that continues to this day. Indeed, AA and other 12-step counseling programs, developed in the 1930s, have a near monopoly on addiction treatment in the United States, with only about 10 percent of rehab clinics offering any evidence-based treatment.

For decades now, the pseudo-religious AA's 12-step approach, emphasizing abstinence and submission to a "creator," has dominated the recovery industry. Historically, then, the treatment of substance or drug-use disorder developed outside mainstream medicine, and today we're still suffering from that.

To be fair to Bill Wilson, he never intended his organization to be twisted into a profitable industry, nor did he ever intend it to be antimedicine. *Alcoholics Anonymous: The Story of How Many Thousands of Men and Women Have Recovered from Alcoholism* (generally known as the Big Book) warns against AA members playing doctor to the detriment of other members. Wilson himself advocated for research into the medical treatment of alcoholism, going as far as beseeching the doctors who created methadone for drug addicts in the 1960s to find a comparable treatment for alcoholics.

Furthermore, until the advent of evidence-based treatment, AA was the only viable alternative for addicts in a society that certainly stigmatized and often criminalized them. AA meetings at least offered safe sanctuary to kindred spirits in a world that truly did not understand them.

The problem with AA originates in its loose structure—it keeps no records and its members are anonymous—and its oblique, often contradictory statements. AA's philosophy could be interpreted and co-opted by anyone. For example, AA's doctrinal Big Book tells us that alcoholism is a disease, yet the treatment it recommends has nothing to do with medicine or science. At best, AA is a kind of spiritually tinged psychological counseling that we call "group therapy" today.

AA also contributed to the stigmatization of the addict and alcoholic thanks to the notion that if its 12-step program doesn't work, it's the fault of the follower, not the program itself. To wit, here's an excerpt from the Big Book: "Rarely have we seen a person fail who has thoroughly followed our path. Those who do not recover are people who cannot or will not completely give themselves to this simple program, usually men and women who are constitutionally incapable of being honest with themselves. They are such unfortunates. They are not at fault; they seem to have been born that way."

In one sense, AA was spot on when it said that addicts "seem to have been born that way." But by mixing that simple statement of fact with pseudo-science, AA planted the roots of today's for-profit rehab industry. AA has become the cover for the highly lucrative nontreatment of addiction in the United States.

The Big Business of Rehab

Make no mistake. Recovery is an industry—a huge business with more than $34 billion in revenue in 2013—and one in which 90 percent of the treatment centers blithely follow and promote the fact their treatment is based on AA's 12-step philosophy. Never mind that even by AA's own admission, only 5 to 8 percent of those who ever attend a single meeting stay sober for more than a year. Indeed, a comprehensive study of treatment programs in the early 2000s, later published as *The Handbook of Alcoholism Treatment Approaches*, ranks AA thirtieth out of forty-eight methods. Just like in *Alice's Adventures in Wonderland*, things happen that do not make any sense and are the opposite of what you would expect.

Why don't all the rehab clinics switch to a scientific treatment of addiction? After all, being profitable and providing effective treatment are not mutually exclusive.

The answer is the degree of profitability. It would greatly

increase the cost of doing business and diminish profits if rehab clinics adopted a scientific approach to treating addiction. Evidence-based medicine must be administered by trained medical professionals. A 12-step program is largely self-administered, costing facilities virtually nothing in labor or, at most, the expense of a low-level addiction counselor—a job that has no mandated requirements (not even a college degree) in most states.

The other reason the vast majority of rehab clinics don't use evidence-based medicine is because they don't have to. There are no federal laws governing what constitutes an addiction treatment center and most state laws are weak and loosely defined. Truly, in most states, you can open a rehab clinic in your living room, call yourself the chief addiction counselor and openly advertise your business with impunity. And, you can shroud the whole farce in the mantle of respectability by trumpeting that you offer AA's 12-step treatment. (AA will never dispute it.)

Unfortunately, this charade is not limited to backyard operations. Two of the most respected names in addiction treatment—the Betty Ford Center, located in southern California and Hazelden Foundation in Minnesota—merged in 2014 into one business venture. In one of his first interviews on the merger with the *Los Angeles Times*, the new CEO of the combined facilities, Mark Mishek, matter-of-factly dismissed evidence-based medicine for addiction treatment. "Nonprofits that have abstinence-based programs that are focused on the 12 Steps of Alcoholics Anonymous need to stick together. We are under attack from a competitive perspective," he said.

Hazelden has a special placeholder in the development of the rehab industry in the United States. In 1949, it was the first center to open using AA's 12 steps as its treatment modality. This in itself was a curious development, because AA founder Bill Wilson purposely created the organization with a bottom-up structure (he called it "benign anarchy"). Individual AA branches were meant to be self-governing. Hazelden turned that notion upside down by establishing a top-down structure and adding discipline to its treatment, in effect, embracing the AA 12 steps without its self-governing philosophy.

Is it any wonder that the public remains confused about addiction when no less than the name of Betty Ford—a former First Lady of the United States who became synonymous with addiction—is evoked to reject modern-day, scientifically proven treatments?

The Problem with AA in the Twenty-First Century

There is no war being fought against AA. Most clinicians, like myself, who deal every day with addicts know that 12-step programs can be a valuable tool in the management of the chronic disease of addiction. Like all chronic diseases, treatment over the long term requires, first, medications and, second, psychological therapy and counseling about lifestyle choices. For some substance abusers, a 12-step program can help them manage their chronic condition.

The problem with AA occurs when it's used instead of or to exclusion of evidence-based medicine. And, while we should point a finger at a rehab industry that preys on some of the most vulnerable in society, AA itself—or, rather, some of its hardcore members—also must share in the blame.

Self-appointed AA sponsors too often demand that those under their supervision renounce all medications, including those helping them with their addiction and, in many cases, a dual diagnosed mental disorder, notably depression. That's not only galling from the perspective of anyone in the medical profession and particularly the field of addiction medicine, it's also dangerous. I've seen too many patients who have suffered serious health consequences—even suicide—after following the advice of a 12-step sponsor to abandon all their medications. While an AA pamphlet states that "No AA members should play doctors; all medical advice and treatment should come from a qualified physician," there is absolutely no consequence if an AA sponsor thumbs her nose at the mandate and demands the new member embrace complete abstinence (meaning no drugs, even medications).

As bad as AA is, its cousin Narcotics Anonymous (NA), whose philosophy incorporates Bill Wilson's 12-step method, is worse. It publicly states it is proudly a "program of abstinence and that a member who takes medication like Suboxone violates the organization's philosophy." In a recent interview with the *Huffington Post*, NA national office's public relations manager Jane Nickels said that if addicts "are taking a drug to treat their addiction, they are not clean in our eyes."

Plenty of Blame to Spread Around

The medical profession itself is also part of the problem. Doctors who don't fully understand the concept of addiction as a chronic disease (with medications available to treat it) are too quick to send a patient who admits to substance abuse to a 12-step program. The prime directive of a doctor is to do no harm to the patient, and such cavalier treatment of patients with a diagnosed alcohol or drug addiction violates this solemn oath. There are too few doctors who have been trained to diagnose and treat addictions. Only 2.5 percent of primary care doctors are certified to prescribe one of the most effective anti-addiction medications, Suboxone.

Like too many doctors, too many judges willfully embrace their ignorance of addiction medicine and send addicts into the hands of 12-step treatment centers, even when evidence-based treatment centers exist as alternatives. Who's to judge whether talking about your problems with other addicts or being treated by a medical professional is the better course of treatment, right?

Private insurance companies and Medicaid also contribute to the problem. In eleven states, Medicaid programs put limits of one to three years on how long addicts can be prescribed Suboxone, one of the leading medications used in addiction treatment. Imagine if we had similar limitations on inhalers for asthma sufferers and insulin for diabetics. The restriction reflects a fundamental misunderstanding that addiction can somehow be cured. Like every other chronic disease (they would not be "chronic" if they could be cured), addiction cannot be cured. But it can be treated and managed successfully so that a high quality of life is achieved.

Some managed care organizations mandate authorization of Suboxone every month. Medicaid has tried to deny payment for Suboxone if a patient fails a drug test. Um, the patient is taking Suboxone to wean himself off a narcotic, so of course it will be present in his body. Equally puzzling, Medicaid will also at times deny payment for Suboxone if the drug test is clean. In other words, you can't win.

If not covered by Medicaid, the Affordable Care Act (ACA), or private insurance, addiction medications can be prohibitively expensive, costing thousands of dollars.

The media, which should be the arbiter of truth, also sometimes gets it all wrong. In a 2013 article sensationally headlined, "Addiction Treatment with a Dark Side," the *New York Times*, no less, asserted that Suboxone was linked to 420 deaths in the United States by the Food and Drug Administration (FDA). The FDA later repudiated the article's false assumption that Suboxone was a cause of the purported overdose deaths and rather was merely detected. The fact of the matter is that, like marijuana, it's almost impossible to overdose on Suboxone.

Finally, blame popular entertainment for creating a narrative spanning decades that the only way to treat substance abuse is through AA. Literally, dozens of films have reinforced this notion, including *Lost Weekend*, circa 1945 with Ray Milland (who won an Oscar for his performance); *Come Back, Little Sheba* (1952, with an Oscar-winning performance by Shirley Booth); *The Days of Wine and Roses* (1962, another Oscar winner; are we seeing a pattern here?); *Clean and Sober* (1988), starring Michael Keaton; *The Basketball Diaries* (1995), starring Leonardo di Caprio; *Leaving Las Vegas* (1995), starring Nicholas Cage (who won an Oscar for his performance) and Elisabeth Shue; *28 Days* (2000), starring Sandra Bullock; *Half Nelson* (2006), starring Ryan Gosling; and on and on.

Of course, many of the films about addiction were made before the advent of evidence-based medicine beginning in the 1990s. Still, having the climax of a film's plotline revolve around a dramatic scene where the protagonist overcomes his addiction through sheer willpower remains very tempting to Hollywood. Treating addiction as a chronic disease through modern science—like hypertension—isn't half as sexy.

The Story of Russell

I am an addiction medicine specialist, psychiatrist, and assistant clinical professor of psychiatry and the behavioral sciences at the University of Southern California. I treat patients, educate medical students, and conduct research.

I wanted to write this book to deliver a clear message: alcoholism and addiction are preventable, treatable medical conditions. But I was motivated to write by a young man I encountered in the ER.

In addition to diagnosing and treating patients, I also provide hands-on education to medical students and doctors in training at Los Angeles County Psychiatric Emergency Services. One evening, I met an emotional and physical wreck of a man brought in by the California Highway Patrol. He had flagged them down on the interstate and begged them to rescue him from the voices in his head and from those pursuing him.

They immediately brought him to the emergency room, and I was promptly notified. I gathered my team of doctors and interns, and we went to the ER to ascertain what was going on. I will never forget what I saw and what I heard from the lips of this most distraught and disheveled young man.

Drenched in sweat, he was a walking nightmare. His clothes were dirty, tattered and torn, and his skin had numerous scrapes and scratches. He was highly agitated, and his eyes darted back and forth as if he were expecting someone to break in at any moment.

We calmly assured him that we were there to help him and that we needed to know how he wound up on the freeway. Despite his extreme agitation, or perhaps because of it, he eagerly poured out his story.

He was a thirty-year-old from Sacramento who had come to Los Angeles for alcohol treatment. He'd been drinking a case of beer and 1.5 liters of vodka every day for the past ten years, and he finally turned to his father for help. He was sent to a free, church-sponsored rehab center in Los Angeles where there was no medical staff awaiting his arrival, no medical diagnosis of his condition, and no medical detox service. All that awaited him was a bed and spiritual counseling.

By the second day in rehab, he had the shakes, anxiety, insomnia, and paranoia—all signs of potentially life-threatening alcohol withdrawal. He asked the resident pastor for help and was given one Tylenol and told to pray.

On the third day, he became further disoriented and even more paranoid. He was hearing voices and having disturbing hallucinations that got worse by the moment. Fearing for his sanity and his life, he made a daring decision. He escaped from the rehab center under the cover of darkness, scaled the chain-link fence and threw himself over the side to the bushes below.

He tore his clothes in the process and sustained numerous scratches and abrasions. Terrified, disoriented, and believing he was being chased by the rehab staff, he struggled through bushes and brambles in almost total darkness before sighting the interstate.

He forced himself over the concrete wall onto the busy freeway, where he dodged traffic until spotted by the highway patrol. He could have been splattered on the interstate or died of seizures in his delirious and psychotic state before being rescued.

We diagnosed his condition as alcohol withdrawal and immediately started him on appropriate medications. His crisis situation was under control within three days, but a CT scan revealed significant brain damage from years of heavy drinking. His brain looked as if it belonged to a demented seventy-year-old.

I arranged a scholarship for him at one of the few medically based treatment centers in the area, and I supervised his medical care personally. He is now independent, working, attending church meetings, and in a happy personal relationship.

Had he not escaped from rehab, he would be dead. He

needed far more than a Tylenol and prayer. I have no problem with prayer. Pray all you want. But I absolutely assure you that whatever benefits prayer may offer are greatly increased when you take the right medicine.

Reality Check: Addiction Treatment Today

This one young man was fortunate that he didn't die from alcohol withdrawal, but others are not so lucky. There are detox places where patients are tied down to a bed and "allowed to detox." If they survive, they are the lucky ones. If not, that's too bad. One of my patients referred to these places as "Deathbed Detox." And they're all legal in the United States.

If you are poor, that is what you can expect in the way of detox and rehab in the progressive and enlightened state of California. Even those who can afford high-priced treatment centers often find themselves in facilities that don't bother to diagnose their medical conditions. The center evaluates insurance but not the patient. It's big business with big profits. Success rates are minimal, even for the most expensive facilities.

While there are a few excellent treatment centers that have full-time medical specialists on staff, most drug and alcohol rehabs do not offer comprehensive medical diagnosis or individualized care.

Just Who Is an Addict?

I began writing this book specifically for individuals concerned about their own relationship to drugs and alcohol or that of someone they love. I wanted to dispel myths, counter outright propaganda, and give people hope where they previously had fear and despair. The more I wrote, the more I realized the importance of reaching the largest audience possible. Too many people believe that anyone who drinks often is an alcoholic and anyone who uses a recreational drug is an addict at worse, drug dependent at best. Those who are *not* addicts are told that they are; those who *are* addicts are being treated with two long-standing failed methods: slogans and stigma.

The probability of becoming an addict is less than the probability of becoming dependent. Your probability of becoming dependent is estimated to be 32 percent for tobacco; 23 percent for heroin; 17 percent for cocaine; 15 percent for alcohol; 11 percent for stimulants other than cocaine; 9 percent for cannabis; 9 percent for anxiolytic, sedative, and hypnotic drugs; 8 percent for analgesics; 5 percent for psychedelics; and 4 percent for inhalants.

A series of studies on the rate of addiction/behavioral dependence in chronic users of nicotine, alcohol, and opioids elegantly demonstrated that only a subpopulation of chronic substance users becomes dependent.

A majority of substance users do not develop addiction. I would venture to say that the majority of people who attend AA meetings and other 12-step programs aren't addicts, either. They may have indulged in heavy drinking or drugging and perhaps at the risk of life and limb to themselves and others (a driving under the influence, DUI, citation is a wake-up call that sends droves of individuals to seek help from AA). And perhaps this is where an AA program excels—that is, facilitating a drinker at risk to examine her bad behavior.

Addicts are different. They suffer from a chronic disease characterized by an inability to abstain from substances they know are harmful. The heavy drinker might down a bottle of vodka while partying into the night. The addict-alcoholic drinks two bottles of vodka or more until he passes out. Addicts can't stop drinking or drugging because their behavioral control—including the ability to stop craving—is impaired.

Those who develop addiction do so primarily because of genetics. The genetic model of addiction predicts that addiction is more likely to develop after initial substance use in individuals with a genetic susceptibility. The more we know about genetics and genetic testing, the more we know about predicting and treating addiction. The addiction is not in the drug; it is in the genes of the individual.

Unfortunately, AA and their allies—most of the rehab industry—don't make those kinds of distinctions. AA true believers actually deny the medical evidence that contradicts their outdated concept of addiction, including that all-or-nothing abstinence is the only hope for recovery. The rehab industry is much more cynical, taking the easy money and using AA's philosophy to rationalize and justify its dismal success rates.

The social stigma of addiction is more destructive in many

cases than the disease itself, and the irresponsible continuation of false diagnoses of addiction by people with no medical credentials, combined with coerced treatment of people for a disease they may not have in the first place, especially when such treatment is devoid of comprehensive medical diagnosis, is an insult to both the patient and the entire medical profession.

Extreme Prejudice

In the all-important, life-saving profession of medicine, we must be clear and precise when discussing addictions. If the general public is wallowing in ignorance, their decisions and actions based on ancient errors and disproved assumptions, illness, and unhappiness will not only continue but increase. No person of good will and integrity would willingly promulgate ignorance.

Superstition is the child of ignorance. In a world of superstition, people believe in magical thinking, distrust new information, and cling tenaciously to outworn and even dangerous practices. A recent guest on a TV talk show insisted, with a perfectly straight face, that there was "real danger" in the practice of yoga because "Hindu demons could take up residence in your spine." Our world is full of people who believe in demons but not in germs, despite overwhelming evidence of germs and none of demons. In this Information Age, the proliferation of misinformation is unparalleled, and erroneous beliefs regarding addiction and treatment are numerous.

One fact is certain: Americans have an extreme prejudice against people suffering from the disease of addiction. This same prejudice is not shown against people with asthma, heart disease, or diabetes, despite these diseases sharing remarkable medical similarities. The reason we fear and distrust addicts is because of their behavior.

Writer and social activist Susan Sontag said it right when she observed about addiction: "Any important malady caused by something obscure and that has an inefficient treatment has the tendency to be full of meaning. At first, the objects of deepest fear (corruption, decadence, pollution, anomie, weakness) are identified with the disease. The disease itself becomes a metaphor. Then, in its name (that is, using it as a metaphor), that horror is imposed on other things. The disease begins to describe things."

Diabetics don't write bad checks to buy Snickers bars, and people with clogged arteries don't break into McDonald's to steal hamburgers. But alcoholics write bad checks to buy more alcohol. The object of addiction takes priority in the damaged decision making of someone with addiction.

Addiction Is Treatable

This is an exciting time in medicine. Astonishing technology allows us to study the actual workings of the human brain, and there are continual breakthroughs in the treatment of chronic illness, including addiction. Researchers are on the cusp of identifying the eleven genes that look to be the hereditary component of addiction.

While scientific treatment of addiction continues to be hobbled by misconceptions and prejudice, there are many glimmers of lights at the end of the tunnel. Remember how Hazelden's CEO touted the virtues of its 12-step program when it merged with the Betty Ford Center in 2014? Well, quietly behind the scenes at the same time, Hazelden's chief medical officer Marvin Seppala was introducing evidence-based medications like Suboxone into its treatment protocols. The results were dramatic. The drop-out rate at Hazelden for opiate addicts in the new medically assisted treatment decreased to just 7 percent compared to 22 percent of those patients not in the new program. In the program's first year, not one addict died from an overdose.

If the two biggest brands in the rehab industry can see the light, change engrained ways, and adopt medically assisted treatment, there's hope for the entire industry.

We must keep in mind, too, that like the privately run healthcare system of the United States, its addiction treatment industry is an anomaly in the world. In every other industrialized nation, addiction is treated like the chronic disease it is. France established evidence-based treatment of addicts in 1995 and saw the country's overdose deaths drop by 79 percent. Similar results have been reported in other Western countries, including Finland, Portugal, Switzerland, and Australia—all places where the grip of the AA philosophy never really took hold like it did in the United States.

Here in America the effectiveness of evidence-based medicine was witnessed in Baltimore with the publicly funded Baltimore Buprenorphine Initiative, which spurred a 50 percent reduction in the city overdose deaths over a fifteen-year period beginning in 1995.

The biggest change in addiction treatment will come when we stop seeing addiction as more of a crime than a disease. Until that time, the treatment of this chronic medical condition will be dominated by misguided amateurs and profiteering rehab providers— who put power and profit over patient well-being.

For the sake of saving lives, we must unite to eliminate prejudice against those born with this genetic predisposition, ensure honest and accurate public education on the subject of addiction, and protect people from fraudulent treatment.

Chapter 2

The Ten Biggest Myths of Addiction

After billions of dollars spent on the disinformation campaign known as the war on drugs, no wonder the American public is confused about alcohol and drug addiction. It's a crime. It's a moral failing. It's the parents' fault. It's the kids' fault.

So, why does it matter? It's important because public perception of alcohol and drugs, their use and abuse, influences public policy. From the length of sentences given to those arrested for possession of various kinds of illicit drugs to the billions of taxpayer dollars spent on addiction treatment, the truth about alcohol and drug addiction has a huge impact on society.

It's also a matter of life and death. Countless addicts are sent by courts—or seek help on their own—at treatment programs where there is no hope for recovery. It's not that real treatment doesn't exist, but rather that most Americans, doctors, judges, and addiction counselors have missed the memo.

The only thing standing between effective treatment of alcohol and drug addiction, based on real medicine, is misinformation and ignorance.

In this chapter I tell it straight—no spin, no hidden agenda, no ulterior motives. Only by telling and absorbing the real facts about alcohol and drug addiction will the American public and its elected leaders be able to come to terms with a rational strategy for dealing effectively with addiction. The truth shall, indeed, set us free.

So, take a walk with me now down the Hall of Shame of the ten biggest myths about alcohol and drug addiction.

1. Addiction Is a Problem of Willpower and Abstinence, Which Is Why Medications Don't Work

The biggest myth of all is that addiction is a problem of willpower and abstinence. The foundation for the sorry state of addiction treatment in this country was inadvertently started in the 1930s by an out-of-work investment banker named Bill Wilson. At the time Wilson had his revelation of what would become Alcoholics Anonymous, he was being treated in a hospital for alcoholism with an experimental drug whose active ingredient was belladonna, a plant known for its hallucinogenic effects (or death, if you ingest too large of a dose). Ironic, isn't it? The man who would set the standard treatment for addiction in the United States in the twenty-first century was being medicated with a psychoactive substance when he came up with it during the Great Depression.

Here's the fact of the matter: There isn't now nor was there ever any evidence that AA's 12-step group talk therapy could treat addiction effectively. Indeed, AA itself never claimed to be the end-all answer to addiction and qualified the idea by emphasizing that its particular pseudo-spiritual philosophy isn't for everyone.

That's not to say that AA 12-step programs cannot be helpful as part of an overall treatment program for addiction that includes medications, psychological counseling, and lifestyle modifications. And by the way, that formula for treatment sounds a lot like the treatment protocol for other chronic brain diseases like bipolar disorder. However, AA is part of the problem of addiction treatment in America because it's remained intransigent on the point that its philosophy of abstinence alone can work miracles.

Fortunately, modern science tells us something different. Through diagnostic tools like MRI, we can see how the brain circuitry of addicts is wired differently from nonaddicts. The advent and use of pharmaceutical drugs since the mid-1990s to stop the craving that is characteristic of substance addiction clearly show us that medications can and do work. Thanks to evidence-based treatment, thousands of addicts formerly debilitated by their disease are living happy and normal lives: holding jobs, paying taxes, and surrounding themselves with friends and family.

2. Addicts Should Be Punished for Using Drugs and Drinking Too Much Because in the End, They Know Better

It is not a crime in the United States to have the physical illness of addiction. But if the object of your addiction, such as illicit drugs, is illegal, you could be arrested and prosecuted for the mere act of possessing it. However, this places the person suffering from addiction in a situation of continually interacting with the criminal underworld rather than with medical professionals.

Imagine if we criminalized insulin or inhalers? Our jails would be filled with diabetics and asthma patients.

U.S. Supreme Court Justice Potter Stewart clearly and eloquently defined the problem in 1962 when he wrote in the case of *Robinson v. California* that "drug addiction is an illness and not a crime" and that "punishing someone for an illness violates the 8th Amendment of the U.S. Constitution."

Let's take it from another perspective. Numerous studies have shown it's much less expensive to treat people with drug problems than to toss them into prison.

Adding to the Alice in Wonderland nature of addiction and criminal law in the United States is the fact that alcohol—*the most* destructive of all addictive drugs in terms of the consequences to the individual and society—is legal, heavily marketed and commercialized, and even glamorized in popular culture.

3. Alcohol Is Different from Other Drugs Because It's Easier to Control and You're Less Likely to Become Addicted to It

Because of our particular culture, we are less harsh on alcoholics than we are on people addicted to other drugs. When we think of heroin addicts, for example, our mental image is *not* one of a charming and upstanding citizen. We think of them as evil, scandalous thieves and criminals. Most people don't know that heroin was once considered a "wonder drug"; it was 100 percent legal and available over the counter.

When heroin was first introduced by Bayer (the same company that gave us aspirin), tuberculosis and pneumonia were the leading causes of death, and even routine coughs and colds could be severely incapacitating. Heroin, which both depresses respiration and gives a restorative night's sleep as a sedative, seemed a godsend. It was used in the treatment of asthma, bronchitis, and tuberculosis and even in the treatment of alcoholism.

According to an article in the *Boston Medical and Surgical Journal* in 1900, "It [heroin] possesses many advantages over morphine. It's not hypnotic, and there's no danger of acquiring a habit." Heroin was widely used in America, and most medicines used by women for relief of menstrual pain contained heroin. Cocaine, a stimulant and anesthetic, was also legal; it was often used in combination with heroin in various medications, often in an alcohol base.

Both heroin and cocaine were inexpensive until they became illegal. Suddenly, the price went sky high, and those already addicted had no choice but to get the money by any means necessary and give that money to criminals.

Alcohol, of course, has long been associated with compulsive, uncontrolled behavior among a certain percentage of the population. The term *alcoholism* was first used in Sweden in 1849, but the first chronicles of uncontrollable urges to drink appear in the early 1800s under the term *dipsomania*. That word actually means compulsive thirst, but it soon became used specifically to mean the compulsive, uncontrolled intake of alcohol.

The classic description of dipsomania was written by Valentin Magnan in 1893, and you will see that he did a very good job of describing what today we call alcoholism:

> Preceded by a vague feeling of malaise . . . dipsomania is a sudden need to drink that is irresistible, despite a short and intense struggle. The crisis lasts from one day to two weeks and consists of a rapid and massive ingestion of alcohol or whatever other strong, excitatory liquid happens to be at hand, whether or not it is fit for consumption. It involves solitary alcohol abuse, with loss of all other interests. These crises recur at indeterminate intervals, separated by periods when the subject is generally sober and may even manifest repugnance for alcohol and intense remorse over his or her conduct. These recurring attacks may be associated with wandering tendencies (dromomania) or suicidal impulses.

Sigmund Freud saw the fevered consumption of alcohol as a complex substitute for sexual obsession and the drunken stupor as a sort of twisted victory in that it successfully desensitized the pain caused by the avoided obsession and featured an alluring mastery of total passivity. Freud considered that motor acts, with or without wandering, were central to sexual obsession, and repetitive drinking was one of those motor skills.

Whether or not Freud's analysis was psychologically accurate, he offered profound insights into the alcoholic's crises. "He never rested until he had lost everything," Freud wrote. "The irresistible nature of the temptation, the solemn resolutions, which are nevertheless invariably broken, never to do it again, the stupefying pleasure and the bad conscience which tells the subject that he is ruining himself (committing suicide)—all these elements remain unaltered in the process."

Freud postulated a hereditary component and delineated similarities between compulsive drinking and compulsive gambling. He also suggested that these compulsions have an association with an organic, toxic brain disease. Decades worth of subsequent research studies have proven him spot-on correct in that regard.

There were early attempts to link alcoholism with manic-depression, now called bipolar disorder, or with a "false manic-depressive" condition. As there were no addiction medicine specialists in those days, there were no empirical medical studies of these conditions beyond noting their characteristics.

Today we know that alcohol is the most prevalent drug abused, causes more deaths than all other drugs combined, and is the most difficult to treat because of its ability to simultaneously affect multiple brain receptors (while other drugs tend to affect only one or two).

4. Virtually Everyone Who Uses Meth or Crack Will Become Addicts and the Meth and Crack Addiction Are Increasing

Most users of meth and crack—like all drugs—never become addicts. Your probability of becoming dependent is estimated to be 32 percent for tobacco; 23 percent for heroin; 17 percent for cocaine and crack; 15 percent for alcohol; 11 percent for stimulants other than cocaine (like meth); 9 percent for cannabis; 9 percent for anxiolytic, sedative, and hypnotic drugs; 8 percent for analgesics; 5 percent for psychedelics; and 4 percent for inhalants. Bottom line: Most people simply stop using their drug of choice before it becomes a real problem.

The misinformation about crack and meth is legion. The very names of these street drugs cause politicians to foam at the mouth. Are they dangerous? Without a doubt. Do they deserve the kind of hysteria they generate? Nope.

It's worth saying again: Most people who try crack don't like it and don't use it again. Over 75 percent of people who tried crack between 2004 and 2006 were not using it at all two years later; 15 percent still smoked it occasionally, but not in a way associated with addiction.

Even though they're the same drug, but in a different form, crack and cocaine are perceived wildly differently both by the criminal justice system and the public alike.

During their lifetime, 7,840,000 (3.3 percent) of Americans have smoked crack cocaine, according to the National Survey on Drug Use and Health. However, only 467,000 (0.2 percent) of Americans reported smoking crack cocaine in the last thirty days. If crack were instantaneously addictive, the number of recent users would be much larger.

According to the same survey of Americans aged twelve and older, 5.9 percent of individuals who had tried cocaine went on to be "current users" (reported use within the past thirty days). The same statistic for crack use was also 5.9 percent. These numbers show no statistical difference in the tendency toward the future use of cocaine and crack.

Again, there is no pharmacological difference between crack cocaine and powder cocaine. Crack cocaine is simply powder cocaine that has been converted into a solid "rock" form that may be smoked. The effects of smoking crack cocaine may be more intense, but this is a result of the mode of ingestion rather than the drug's purity. Regardless, it is difficult to rationalize the extreme sentencing disparity between crack and cocaine.

Similarly, crack is perceived not only to be more addictive but more deadly. The misuse of any drug (legal or illegal) can be detrimental to your health. However, it is simply not true to claim that crack cocaine is a major cause of death. The percentage of deaths attributed to *all* illegal drugs combined is less than 1 percent. By comparison, over 18 percent is caused by tobacco. More people die every year from legal drugs, legally prescribed, than all illegal drugs combined.

Fact: While often characterized as a drug of the black community, 60 percent of individuals who have used crack in the last month are white. White crack users also account for 66 percent of individuals who have ever used crack in their lifetime. Simply stated, the majority of crack users are white.

Despite this reality, 80 percent of people arrested for crack offenses are black. Consequently, a disproportionate number of black crack offenders face the harsh mandatory minimums associated with crack convictions.

Finally, crack is perceived as instigating violent behavior while cocaine gets a pass. Yet, research has shown that crack use does not result in violent behavior. The violence one associates with crack is not from the effects of the drug, but rather the violence between rival criminal organizations and/or law enforcement.

Like crack and cocaine, meth is perceived as a drug with no redeeming value. That's true. About a hundred years ago the same argument was used to ban and criminalize the use of alcohol. What is *not* true is that meth is on the rise and meth users are harder to treat than, say, alcoholics.

Meth use in the United States peaked at least two decades ago and has slightly declined or stayed about the same. Addiction to methamphetamine is not much different from that of any other drug addiction except tobacco, which is the most addicting and the most difficult to quit. When it comes to successful treatment, it doesn't matter if you're talking about meth or heroin or alcohol.

Just as the vast majority of drinkers are not alcoholics, the majority of stimulant users (like meth heads) are not addicts. They stop on their own or with help from family and friends. There is that small minority of those who actually have the disease of addiction and require true medical treatment. These are the people with whom I am concerned.

"Meth is a real problem for some people, but it is an over-hyped problem. All you have to do is look at the use rates and look at sentencing," said Jason Ziedenberg, executive director of the Justice Policy Institute. "When 100,000 people a year die from alcohol, I'm still saying that's the most dangerous drug in America."

5. People Addicted to One Drug Are Addicted to All of Them

It is not true that a person who is addicted to one drug is addicted to all drugs. The drug to which someone becomes addicted corresponds to that individual's particular brain chemistry. Most alcoholics are not meth heads, most heroin junkies don't regularly use meth, and so on. Now, when the preferred drug of choice is scarce (meaning, expensive) or not available at all, addicts will turn to another drug. Read on.

6. Prescription Pills Are Safer Than Illegal Street Drugs Because They've Been Prescribed by a Doctor

The Centers for Disease Control and Prevention (CDC) recently released some startling facts about drug use and deaths in the United States.

- In 2013, of the 43,982 drug overdose deaths in the United States, 22,767 (51.8 percent) were related to pharmaceuticals, notably opioid analgesics (also called prescription painkillers), stimulants, and tranquilizers.
- In 2011, about 1.4 million emergency room (ER) visits involved the nonmedical use of pharmaceuticals. Among those ER visits, 501,207 were related to antianxiety and insomnia medications, and 420,040 were related to opioid analgesics.
- The drug overdose death rate has more than doubled

from 1999—about the same time that doctors dramatically increased the prescribing of painkillers—through 2013.

- In 2013, more than 17,000 people died from prescription painkiller overdoses, with more than 400,000 going to an emergency room.

The CDC called the prescription painkiller epidemic that took hold in the late 1990s the worst of its kind in U.S. history. "The bottom line is that this is one of the few health problems in this country that's getting worse," CDC director Tom Frieden told the *Huffington Post* in 2014.

Echoing those sentiments, the editorial board of *USA Today* wrote in November 2013, "The deadliest drug problem in America is not heroin or cocaine or even crack cocaine. It's the abuse of perfectly legal prescription pain medications—familiar names such as Vicodin and Lortab and generic hydrocodone."

The extent of the prescription pill problem is reflected in this startling statistic: The painkiller hydrocodone is the most prescribed medication in America—136.7 million prescriptions a year at last count. To frame the problem another way, in 2010, enough prescription painkillers were prescribed to medicate every American adult every four hours for one month.

In 2014 the Food and Drug Administration (FDA) and the Drug Enforcement Agency (DEA) began a joint effort to crack down on the prescription pill epidemic by reclassifying hydrocodone, Vicodin, and other leading painkillers in the category reserved for medical substances with the highest potential for harm. The initiative also required patients to present to a pharmacist in person with a written prescription from a qualified health provider—a move to stem the practice of faxing or calling in the prescription multiple times to multiple pharmacies.

The good news is that all of that worked. The tidal wave of prescription pills available on the legal and illegal markets began to recede. The bad news is that pill addicts switched their drug of choice to an equally dangerous drug—heroin.

7. Today's Marijuana Is Extremely Powerful and a Leading Cause of Drug Overdose, thus Possession in Small Amounts Shouldn't Be Decriminalized or Legalized

I could write a book about marijuana myths alone, but I'll confine myself to two points. First, even today with some states legalizing marijuana for personal recreational use, there has not been one recorded death from marijuana overdose. While tens of thousands of people die each year from alcohol or prescription painkillers, no one has ever died or overdosed on marijuana. Why? Let me quote the National Cancer Institute: "Because cannabinoid receptors, unlike opioid receptors, are not located in the brainstem areas controlling respiration, lethal overdoses from Cannabis and cannabinoids [marijuana] do not occur."

Although painkillers can cause a person to stop breathing, you could smoke or ingest marijuana all day and all night and your respiration would still not be affected because marijuana does not affect the body's brain pathway that controls it.

Second, there is no evidence that decriminalizing, legalizing, or otherwise making marijuana more available to the public in any way increases its use. In fact, according to a recent national school-based survey among teens in grades eight through twelve, the increased availability of marijuana in the twenty-one states that legalized medical marijuana did not significantly change its use. The study was conducted by researchers at Columbia University Mailman School of Public Health and supports a growing body of evidence that making legalized marijuana more available to the public does not increase its use.

All this said, I still support the regulation of marijuana. At the moment, there are no federal standards regarding dosages. The problem of nonstandardized packaging—including the lack of clear warning labels—is particularly egregious with marijuana-infused edibles as well as drinks and pills. Unlike smoking a joint, the user can consume a relatively large quantity of THC, the high-inducing compound in marijuana, by eating a cookie, for example. This can impair the user's cognitive and motor skills, a potentially fatal scenario if it involves driving a car.

Ingesting too much THC can also increase the risk of mental illness. Too many people are ending up in the ER for THC-induced intoxication and panic attacks. Unregulated THC-infused products pose an even bigger danger for those at risk of serious mental disorders. A recent study published in the British journal *Psychiatry* showed that large doses of THC can trigger schizophrenia in predisposed patients.

Finally, isn't it obvious to all concerned that edibles such as brownies, cookies, and candy infused with mega doses of THC pose still another danger to children? We regulate alcohol and

The Ten Biggest Myths of Addiction   41

cigarettes, which like marijuana are legalized recreational drugs intended for adult use, with standardized dosages and packaging. Why not, then, marijuana?

8. Heroin Is Mainly a Ghetto Drug

A comprehensive study called, appropriately, "The Changing Face of Heroin Use in the United States," published in 2014 by the journal *JAMA Psychiatry,* reported that contrary to popular belief, most heroin addicts today did not start on their "silk road" to perdition with another illicit drug, such as marijuana. Instead, most first started getting high with prescription painkillers, likely obtained at home, from a friend, or illegally on the street.

As mentioned earlier, the campaign to restrict prescription painkillers simply switched the addiction problem in the United States to heroin, which, unfortunately, at the same time was becoming cheap and plentiful on the black market due to overproduction in the narcotic countries, notably Afghanistan but also Mexico and countries in South America and southeast and southwest Asia.

Quite suddenly, the new prescription painkiller epidemic transformed into the new heroin epidemic. As *The Atlantic* magazine noted in an October 2014 article, "ten years after prescription painkiller dependence" swept America and "the government cracked down on doctors and drug companies, people went searching for a cheaper, more accessible high. Now, many areas are struggling with an unprecedented heroin crisis."

Heroin, the drug that was once exclusively associated with

urban America and particularly black ghettos, was now becoming a fixture in white suburbia and in rural states. The problem became so alarming that in Vermont, everyone's ideal of pastoral beauty in America (not to mention the headquarters of Ben & Jerry's ice cream), the governor devoted his entire annual speech in 2014 to what he called "a full-blown heroin crisis" gripping his state.

In a 2014 article headlined "Heroin Overdose Deaths Quadruple over Last Decade, As Painkillers Open Fatal Gateway," the website Medical Daily reported that the death rate jumped from 0.7 deaths per 100,000 people in the year 2000 to 2.7 deaths per 100,000 in 2013. More troubling, between 2010 and 2013, the death rate made even greater leaps: from a 6 percent increase over the previous decade to 37 percent. "Beneath this trend lurks a more fundamental change in how heroin is used, and, importantly, who is using it. The demographics of fatal overdose have changed considerably in the last decade. In 2000, black adults between forty-five and sixty-four years old showed the highest rate, at two deaths per 100,000. In 2013, white adults between eighteen and forty-four earned that distinction, at seven deaths per 100,000. Some suggest heroin's vanishing stigma can explain the change," according to the report.

Fueling the epidemic was a new, more pure and potent form of heroin that could be snorted or smoked to achieve the high previously possible only through injections. So, while we're at it, let's destroy the other myth about opioids as largely a drug of choice of young people. As it turns out, prescription pill addiction skews much older than other drug epidemics. In 2012, those between the ages of forty-five and sixty-four accounted for the highest rate of inpatient hospital stays for opioid overuse. Two decades earlier, according to the federal Agency for Healthcare Research and Quality, the highest rate was for those between twenty-five and forty-four.

When the supply of prescription pills tightened because of new federal restrictions, baby boomers turned to, yes, marijuana (did they ever leave it?), but right behind it as the most common illegal drug of choice was, according to the National Institutes of Health, heroin (in its new, noninjectable form).

9. Alcoholics and Addicts Have to Hit Rock Bottom before They Can Be Treated Effectively

The need to hit rock bottom is another pseudo-science precept of AA, which, however, welcomes alcoholics to join at any stage of their addiction. Yet, if you're around anyone who is a member of AA, the idea of hitting rock bottom is thrown around like a badge of honor.

There is no medical science that supports the idea that addiction can be treated only once you've blacked out on Skid Row, driven a car into a tree, ended up in a hospital or jail cell, or any other calamities associated with hitting rock bottom. That's tantamount to saying a diabetic can be treated effectively only once he or she goes into insulin shock. It's always better with any chronic disease—be it asthma, heart disease, bipolar diseases, or substance addiction—to get help early. In short, the whole idea of rock bottom is utter nonsense.

How did we reach the point where the treatment of a chronic

disease includes the notion of rock bottom? Part of the reason lies in the origins of AA. Its founder, Bill Wilson, indeed had lost everything of value to him and was hospitalized because of medical conditions related to his illness when he says that he received his epiphany to begin AA. His plight became the model for all AA followers.

Another reason is the double-speak world of AA dogma. *Rock bottom* provides cover for when AA members fall off the wagon. AA can say that its prescribed abstinence-only treatment did not work on those who left because those quitters hadn't yet—and here it comes—hit rock bottom. In the world of AA, the program is never the problem; relapse is always the member's fault.

10. Treating Addiction with Medications Won't Work Because You're Just Substituting One Drug for Another, and Besides, Addicts Will Figure Out a Way to Abuse the New Drug

Recent scientific research shows that the process of addiction is related to overstimulation of the brain's reward pathway. A study published in *Science Daily* states that what happens in addiction to drugs is lethally simple: "The reward pathways in the brain have been so over-stimulated that the system basically turns on itself, adapting to the new reality of addiction, whether it's cocaine or cupcakes."

From a medical perspective, then, the key to treating addiction is crystal clear: Stop the overstimulation of the brain's reward pathway. This is where AA and 12-step programs confuse correlation with cause. Abstinence can be achieved when proper medical treatment is provided, which halts the addict's craving for his favored substance. But simply talking about stopping the craving and listening to stories of other people's addiction will not achieve abstinence for most people.

Modern medical science has given us an array of pharmaceutical medications that have proven effective in stopping the craving that characterizes addiction. We'll get into that deeper in the next chapter, but suffice to say that among the most effective treatments for addiction to opioids (prescription pills, heroin, morphine) is buprenorphine, an FDA-approved, opioid-derived medication. When a patient switches from his opioid of choice to buprenorphine, the addictive behavior usually stops. That's because buprenorphine's ability to cause a high has a ceiling. Patients can snort, smoke, or inject buprenorphine all they want, but extra doses will not make them feel any differently.

Some addicts stay on buprenorphine for weeks or months, others for years. There is no one-size-fits-all cure for addiction. It's a complex disease requiring individualized treatment. Buprenorphine has allowed addicts to live a normal life by helping them regain control of their brain's reward pathways.

I'll close this chapter by acknowledging that buprenorphine is now one of the most sought-after drugs on the streets . . . but not for the reason you might think.

The medication, often dispensed under its brand name Suboxone, is tightly controlled and must be prescribed by a physician specifically trained and licensed to handle the drug. A mere 2.5 percent of all primary care doctors are certified.

As reported in the *Huffington Post* in a 2015 groundbreaking article about the lack of evidence-based treatment ("Dying to Be Free" by Jason Cherkis), multiple states are struggling to manage the heroin epidemic in which "thousands of addicts have no access to Suboxone. There have been reports by doctors and clinics of waiting lists for the medication in Kentucky, Ohio, central New York and Vermont, among others." In one Ohio county, a clinic's waiting list ran to 500 patients.

To be clear, Suboxone has been so effective in dealing with prescription painkiller and heroin addiction that there is a great demand for it by addicts. When addicts can't get it legally, they turn to the black market. As I said before, America doesn't have so much an addiction problem as a problem with addiction treatment.

Chapter 3

The Medical Illness of Addiction

Joanne Campbell, forty-five, is not your idea of an addict. She is a mother with three gainfully employed and happy adult children. She is also a successful retail entrepreneur.

Born in Houston, she was a typical teenager but maybe atypical in that she rarely indulged in drinking or drugging. When she turned twenty-one, the legal drinking age in the state, she started social drinking with friends. She married and, together with her husband, began raising a family.

That's when she discovered cocaine and, by the age of twenty-eight, she was abusing it. She and her spouse split, and she was left to raise her three children on her own. "After my split with the father of my children in 2000 is when I began to abuse alcohol more often," she says.

Over the next decade she recalls that her abuse of cocaine led her to something more serious. "I think that I became addicted over a period of years with the misuse and abuse of alcohol," she says. "It kind of went up and down from the age of 35 to 43. I had some bad years and some fine years, leading up to a couple of really bad years where so many things seemed so overwhelming that I would drink more often and for longer periods of time. I believe that so many emotionally difficult things in my life built up that I had never really dealt with."

It was shortly after Christmas 2011 that Joanne came to see me. Alone at home during the holidays, her three adult children busy with their own lives, she began a familiar routine—a binge of cocaine and alcohol, except this time it didn't stop. When her concerned children finally showed up on her doorstep and gave her an ultimatum, she knew that she had to get help.

Her fear of losing everything, including her children, finally became a reality. For many years, she thought she could do it on her own. At a certain point she even began to see a therapist weekly and thought that she would be able to fix herself through counseling alone.

She had tried AA and 12-step programs but never identified with them. "I think that was also part of my problem," she said. "I didn't think anything else was available."

Realizing the gravity of Joanne's deteriorating health, her therapist recommended that she consider an evidence-based treatment under my medical supervision. After a successful detox, Joanne began a program that managed her addictive cravings through a combination of pharmaceutical intervention and cognitive behavioral therapy (CBT).

Three years later, she is flourishing, running a small business.

She still regularly sees me for management of her addiction disease, but has not relapsed since.

———

Alcohol and drug addiction is a chronic disease with a strong genetic predisposition. Does that sound familiar? It should, because it basically describes every other leading chronic disease, including heart disease, stroke, cancer, diabetes, and asthma. It's also like mental illness because, in addition, addiction is a brain disease.

Addicts and alcoholics have structural or functional damage to the reward-motivation center of their brains. When damaged, this reward center keeps individuals doing things even when the result is pain instead of pleasure.

Whenever you do something pleasurable, it affects the amount of a substance in the brain called dopamine. If there were a pleasure impact scale based on dopamine, eating food and drinking water rates a 2, sex rates 4, cocaine rates 8, and methamphetamine scores a 12.

It's interesting to note that both methamphetamine and cocaine increase the amount of dopamine in the synapses. However, cocaine achieves this action by preventing dopamine reuptake, while methamphetamine helps the body release more dopamine. So although these drugs have similar effects, they work in entirely different ways.

Bottom line: Addiction is a medical condition, not a moral failing. The seemingly age-old debate over the treatment of alcohol and drug addiction—through willpower, spirituality, and talk therapy versus physical diagnosis and evidence-based therapy—is over. The connection between addiction and brain chemistry is indisputable. While there is a role for behavioral and cognitive counseling in addiction treatment, a program based purely on psychological therapy or the 12-step philosophy is inadequate for treating a disease with genetic and physiological roots.

The Anatomy of Addiction

Substance addictions, including alcohol and stimulant drugs like cocaine, are not caused by the drink or the drug. Addiction is primarily the result of genetics and overstimulation of the pleasure and reward pathway in the brain.

In the case of Joanne for example, it was very clear to me when I first diagnosed her that she was motivated to stop drinking. She loved her children, she wanted to pursue her dream of owning her own business, and she knew that she had the skills to turn her life around. But she couldn't stop her craving for alcohol and cocaine. "My addiction would get better for months at a time," Joanne confessed, "but I would always go back to an alcohol and drug binge when I needed to check out of my world."

We now know why the Joannes of the world cannot help themselves. Addiction is a disease characterized by anatomical and functional changes in the human brain. The anatomical changes can be clearly seen and studied with brain imaging technology, such as a standard MRI and CT scans. Functional abnormalities can be seen, studied, and evaluated by PET scans or functional MRI. These changes are in the brain's reward, motivation, memory, and related circuitry. Some of these changes are repairable, while others are not reversible—so far.

Just as heart disease causes a blatantly decreased heart

metabolism, drug abuse causes a similar decrease in brain metabolism. The similarities between addiction and heart disease, diabetes, and asthma are remarkable. They each have a genetic basis and are impacted by voluntary behavior.

Because the brain controls behavior, a disease of the brain will have behavioral consequences. Because of these brain changes, people become unable to make conscious decisions in their own best interest. Individuals thus afflicted with the disease will compulsively pursue a detrimental course of action, despite continual negative medical and social consequences. In other words, despite knowing that the next bottle of vodka that he consumes will likely kill him, especially if he gets behind the wheel of car to go buy it, an alcoholic will quite literally drive himself to drink.

About 10 percent of the at-risk population becomes alcoholics or drug addicts—and the rest do not. Let's reframe that: Most people who drink alcohol, snort cocaine, or shoot heroin will not become addicts. Why? Research indicates that fully half the reason is genetic. For instance, we know that the children of alcoholics are four to five times more likely to become alcoholics themselves.

The exact mechanisms of how drugs and alcohol affect the addict's brain are still being worked out. But we know a lot right now. We know that alcohol and drugs in everyone's brains affect the delicate equilibrium in the neurological system. Pulses travel along this network of nerves, carrying information and instructions from the brain to the rest of the body. Substances called neurotransmitters keep our bodies functioning, from our most fundamental tasks, such as breathing and eating, to more intricate processes like pleasure seeking (including falling in love) and the fight-or-flight response (it's why we automatically jump away from oncoming traffic).

The neurobiology of addiction is very complex, but it appears from numerous studies that two neurotransmitters are especially important in alcohol and drug addiction: GABA and dopamine. GABA is among a group of inhibitory neurotransmitters that regulate and moderate impulses. Dopamine is on the opposite end of the spectrum and belongs to those excitatory neurotransmitters that provide the reward of pleasure. In proper balance, these neurotransmitters allow one to lead a productive and happy life, but without going overboard on the happy part.

In other words, together these two neurotransmitters achieve the moderation that philosophers have extolled through the ages. (The Greek sage Epictetus was among the first to observe, "If one oversteps the bounds of moderation, the greatest pleasures cease to please.")

Even for the normal person, drugs change the brain just like they change the brain of the addict. Psychoactive drugs artificially overstimulate dopamine flow and block the flow of the inhibitory agents in GABA. Forget the stoic advice of Epictetus. Suddenly the brain goes totally Oscar "Nothing succeeds like excess" Wilde.

But eventually, the inhibitory neurotransmitters of the normal person's brain put the brakes on the overstimulation of dopamine, and the person stops drinking or drugging. Those brakes don't work in the addict's brain. They were made defective or they've burned out. And even worse, the more they drink and drug excessively, the more they desensitize the brain's receptors.

Is There an Addiction Gene?

I was interviewed by ABC News when the Oscar-winning actor Robert Downey Jr. appeared on the cover of Vanity Fair *magazine. In the accompanying magazine article, Downey talked about his concern of passing his addictive personality on to his son Indio. (You might also recall that Indio was arrested for cocaine possession in October 2014.)*

I agreed that Downey was correct in believing that genes played a role in addiction, but his son's use of cocaine did not mean he was necessarily going to be an addict. Most teenagers abuse drugs—it is part of growing up in an individualistic culture like America, whether or not parents like it.

Decades of scientific research have shown that the chance of becoming an addict is at least 50 percent—and perhaps as high as 75 percent— the result of your genes. Now, that's not to say that every child of an addict will be one as well. Both clinically and statistically, we know that not to be the case. It does mean, however, that children of addicts have a higher risk, and knowing this can empower them to make lifestyle choices that can help them reduce the risk of getting the disease or controlling it.

There's no good biomarker at the moment to determine if someone is genetically programmed for addiction, so we must rely on behavior and diagnostic tools like MRI and behavioral analysis to make a predictive determination (more on this in Chapter 5). But what if a gene

for addiction were identified that then could be manipu-
lated so that the disease could be avoided altogether?

Researchers are zeroing in on the genetic basis for
drug and alcohol addiction. The National Institutes of
Health, the National Institute on Alcohol Abuse and
Alcoholism, and the National Institute on Drug Abuse all
have studies under way that seek to explain the effects of
alcohol and stimulant drugs by identifying specific genes
that may be predictive of use as well as shed light on any
underlying molecular or behavioral factors involved.

New research indicates that there isn't just one "addiction gene" but rather a panel of five to eleven genes associated with alcohol and drug abuse. Investigators at Indiana
University have published results of a study that asks, if an
individual is found to have the genetic predisposition across
these eleven genes, is he or she predestined to be—or at
least, at very high risk—of being an addict? Stay tuned.

Other research is focused on the *epigenetics* of drug
addiction, meaning how use, and particularly high volume use, over a long term actually alters the structure of
DNA. Most of our DNA is locked in when we're born,
but not completely. Environmental factors—ranging from
exposure to radiation to everyday stress—can have lasting effects on body and brain functions.

In a study at the University of California at San Fran-
cisco, scientists found that long-term alcohol abuse changes
the chemical signatures around specific genes that shield
against addiction. Once changed, these protective systems never return to their full effect. As the researchers
explained, this mechanism might help explain "as to why

10 percent of the population develops alcohol use disorders" and why the rest of population that indulges alcohol does not.

In other words, neuroscience is showing us that the basis of drug and alcohol abuse is found in both a pattern of genes causing risky behavior and also a pattern of risky behavior that changes the way our genes are expressed.

Why is this important? First, if a person knows definitively—beyond his familial history—that he has a genetic profile for addiction, he can take proactive steps to avoid the kind of behavior that would trigger the disease (like, for instance, avoiding alcohol and recreational drugging).

Second, knowing the genetic and epigenetic basis for addiction could be extremely helpful in the development of future medications to treat and even prevent addiction.

Finally, the emerging technique of gene therapy, which uses specific genes to treat or prevent disease, is on the cusp of entering mainstream medicine. What if in the not too distant future, doctors could treat an alcohol or drug disorder by inserting a gene into the patient's cells to correct the faulty brain circuitry that characterizes addicts? This level of understanding might even lead to the elusive cure for the chronic disease of addiction.

A New Normal

Addicts develop a "new normal" because the brain attempts to adjust to the foreign substances—the toxins—flooding its receptors. Eventually, every addict reaches a tipping point, where the brain receptors remain permanently on. The first puff of marijuana or snort of heroin can send the addict back to the level of addiction when she hit bottom.

That likely is what happened with Oscar-winning actor Philip Seymour Hoffman, who died of a heroin overdose. He admitted quite openly during his career that as a young man he tried every drug that he could get his hands on, not to mention alcohol. His official death, at age forty-six, was ruled as acute mixed-drug intoxication, including heroin, cocaine, benzodiazepines, and amphetamines. Even though he claimed twenty years of sobriety, three months before his death he purportedly snorted a line of heroin at a party, and it was like nothing had ever changed—he was back in an instant to the addiction that he had experienced as a young man.

Not only does overstimulation of the reward circuitry factor significantly in addiction but it also creates false memories of the experience. The brain regards the experience as "better than expected," even when the experience wasn't all that great. Because the memory is a permanent part of your mental makeup, anything and everything that reminds you of that memory also reminds you that the experience was better than expected and triggers an instant desire to reexperience something that perhaps wasn't anywhere as good as you remember.

Sound twisted and illogical? Well, it is! Welcome to the world of addicts and alcoholics who, no matter how bright they are, rely on a brain that is constantly giving them false signals.

However, an addict doesn't even have to ingest a substance to flip the trigger. An alcoholic can pass a bar and the mere association of the booze inside can create a cascade of anxiety that mimics the feelings of withdrawal. That's why many drug addicts and alcoholics relapse. The craving never disappears. It's always there. It's like every other chronic disease in the sense that the disease is never cured.

The difference between addiction and most other chronic diseases is that it affects the brain. That's important because, as previously mentioned, the brain controls behavior, so a disease of the brain will have behavioral consequences. Because of these brain changes, people become unable to make conscious decisions in their own best interest. The medically accepted definition of addiction clearly states that the individual thus afflicted will compulsively pursue a detrimental course of action, despite continual negative health and social consequences.

Once the brain change has taken place, medical treatment coupled with intentional behavior modification can help restore balance, and in some cases, actually repair damage to the brain's reward circuitry. To make things really clear, here is a useful, if perhaps an oversimplified, formula:

$$GP + ES = A$$

Genetic predisposition (*GP*) + Excessive stimulation of the pleasure–reward pathway (*ES*) = Addiction (*A*)

Therefore, for someone with a genetic predisposition to addiction, an effective preventive measure is a diversity of pleasures, none of them to excess. Knowing that too much pleasure repeated too often, especially from a singular source, is a major factor in addiction, the wise person practices moderation, enjoys a variety of different activities, and guards against overdoing any one thing.

Addiction is characterized by the inability to consistently abstain, by impairment in behavioral control, by cravings, by diminished recognition of significant problems with one's behaviors and interpersonal relationships, and by a dysfunctional emotional response. Like other chronic diseases, addiction often involves cycles of relapse and remission. Without treatment or engagement in recovery activities, addiction is progressive and can result in disability or premature death.

With addiction, there is a significant impairment in executive functioning (the part of the brain that organizes and acts on information), which manifests in problems with perception, learning, impulse control, compulsivity, and judgment. People with addiction often manifest a lower readiness to change their dysfunctional behaviors, despite mounting concerns expressed by significant others in their lives. They also display an apparent lack of appreciation of the magnitude of cumulative problems and complications.

The still developing frontal lobes of adolescents, in particular, may both compound these deficits in executive functioning and predispose youngsters to engage in high-risk behaviors, including alcohol or other drug use. The profound drive or craving to use substances or engage in apparently rewarding behaviors underscores the compulsive aspect of this disease. This is the connection with "powerlessness" over addiction and "unmanageability" of life, as is described in the first step of 12-step programs.

The Effects of Alcohol on the Brain

It's at this point where we must stop thinking of drug and alcohol addiction as synonymous. In terms of its physiological effect on the body and its consequences to the health of the addict, alcohol is much more insidious and its damage more serious.

Despite alcohol consumption being both socially acceptable and perfectly legal, it kills more people than any other drug in the United States. Alcohol is the third leading cause of death, because it attacks every vital organ system in the human body. Yet, the fact that it is legal—even celebrated and glamorized—makes it far more acceptable than, say, crack in modern society. Keep in mind that at the advent of the twentieth century both cocaine and heroin were sold as over-the-counter medications, and wealthy white women were more likely to be addicted to drugs, including morphine, than any other group in the country. (Celebrated early twentieth-century American playwright Eugene O'Neill made repeated references to his mother's morphine addiction in plays such as *Long Day's Journey into Night*.)

The physical effects of alcohol addiction are far more widespread than addiction to drugs. Alcohol directly or indirectly causes stomach cancer, rectum cancer, colon cancer, throat cancer, liver cancer, larynx cancer, and esophageal cancer. Alcohol doesn't cause lung cancer, but as many alcoholics also smoke, you might take that into consideration as well.

Scientists used to think of alcohol as a membrane disruptor with a generalized effect all over the brain, as the small molecule can freely diffuse across the blood–brain barrier. We now know that there are particular cells in the brain that alcohol targets by binding certain hydrophobic pockets on their surface receptors.

Unlike opioids (heroin, opium, morphine, oxycodone, and Vicodin), which tend to affect only one kind of cellular receptor, alcohol has been found to affect more than 100 unique receptors in the brain. It activates the entire neurotransmitter reward system.

The neurochemical effects of alcohol cause a range of short-term effects—from a mild buzz to slow reaction times, which make drunk driving so dangerous. In the long term, these effects are also the basis for two of the defining characteristics of alcoholism: *tolerance* and *dependence*.

Tolerance to alcohol is one aspect of alcoholism that leads to overdrinking. Tolerance can be acute, in one bout of drinking, or long-term, requiring an ever-larger dose to get the same effect over time.

The effect of acute tolerance is a common experience for anyone who has had more than a few drinks. Initially, the first drink has a relaxing effect, but as a person continues drinking, it takes more and more alcohol to produce the same effect. Some people have more acute tolerance than others due to genetic factors. These are the people who can drink everyone else under the table, and they also may be at increased risk of developing dependence on alcohol.

Dependence on alcohol is linked to the interaction of alcohol with the brain's stress system, which alcohol activates. The major component of the brain's stress system is corticotropin-releasing factor (CRF) in the amygdala and related areas, which activates sympathetic and behavioral responses to stress. In a normal stress response, CRF recruits other parts of the brain to help adapt the mind and body to deal with the physical and mental stressors that challenge it. Alcohol interacts in such a way as to acutely reduce CRF levels in the brain; chronic alcoholism does the opposite.

Research indicates that individuals who are at increased risk of becoming alcoholics are likely to have a genetic makeup causing them to have higher CRF levels than normal. They may be drinking to tame a hyperactive CRF stress system in the brain.

Unfortunately, CRF and the stress system adjust to the alcohol. In the absence of alcohol, the alcoholic feels ill because his or her body cannot easily reverse the high levels of CRF and low reward neurotransmission. This ill feeling may contribute to the tendency of the alcoholic to overdrink—a danger because of the toxic effect on the brain and body of subjecting oneself to so much alcohol.

Sadly, the brain often does not perceive the consequences of the short-term relief that the alcohol brings. When a person over-drinks, she feels good while she is boozing. However, this short-term relief makes the whole system worse off.

Not Either/Or, but Both

During the last century, a debate raged in academic circles whether addiction was a psychological disorder or a physiological disease. Was it a behavioral problem that arises because of environmental factors in early childhood—the nurture argument? Or was addiction a hereditary disease—the nature argument?

We now know it's both. Addiction is a disease with a strong genetic component that also includes aspects of behaviors, cognitions, emotions, and interactions with others, including the addict's ability to relate to members of her family, to members of her community, to her own psychological state, and to things that transcend her daily experience.

Behavioral manifestations and complications of addiction, primarily due to impaired control, can include the following:

- Excessive use and/or engagement in addictive behaviors at higher frequencies and/or quantities than the person intended, often associated with a persistent desire for and unsuccessful attempts at behavioral control.

- Excessive time lost in substance use or recovering from the effects of substance use and/or engagement in addictive behaviors, with significant adverse impact on social and occupational functioning (for example, the development of interpersonal relationship problems or the neglect of responsibilities at home, school, or work).

- Continued use and/or engagement in addictive behaviors, despite the presence of persistent or recurrent physical or psychological problems that may have been caused or exacerbated by substance use and/or related addictive behaviors.

- A narrowing of the behavioral repertoire focusing on rewards that are part of the addiction and an apparent lack of ability and/or readiness to take consistent action toward change, despite recognition of problems.

Over time, repeated experiences with substance use or addictive behaviors damage the brain's reward circuit activity and are no longer as subjectively rewarding. Once a person experiences withdrawal from drug use or comparable behaviors, there is an anxious, agitated, and unstable emotional experience related to suboptimal reward and the recruitment of brain and hormonal stress systems, which is associated with withdrawal from virtually all pharmacological classes of addictive drugs.

While tolerance develops to the high, tolerance does not develop to the emotional low associated with the cycle of intoxication and withdrawal. Thus, in addiction, people repeatedly attempt to create a high. But what they mostly experience is a deeper and deeper low. While anyone may *want* to get high, those with addiction feel a *need* to use the addictive substance or engage in the addictive behavior to try to resolve their uncomfortable emotional state or their physiological symptoms of withdrawal. People with addiction compulsively use even though it may not make them feel good.

It is important to appreciate that addiction is not solely—and mostly isn't—a function of choice. Addiction is not a desired condition. Remember what Joanne told us earlier in the chapter? She wanted to stop. She was aware that she should stop. She had every incentive to stop for the sake of her family and her career. But she could not stop—at least not until she was successfully treated. Simply put, people may choose to get high or drunk but no one chooses to be a junkie or an alcoholic.

Abuse vs. Addiction

The terms abuse *and* addiction *have been defined and redefined over the years. The 1957 World Health Organization Expert Committee on Addiction-Producing Drugs defined addiction as:*

> A state of periodic or chronic intoxication produced by the repeated consumption of a drug (natural or synthetic). Its characteristics include: (i) an overpowering desire or need (compulsion) to continue taking the drug and to obtain it by any means; (ii) a tendency to increase the dose; (iii) a psychic (psychological) and generally a physical dependence on the effects of the drug; and (iv) detrimental effects on the individual and on society.

In 1964, a new World Health Organization (WHO) committee found this definition to be inadequate and suggested using the blanket term *drug dependence* instead of drug addiction.

In 2001, the American Academy of Pain Medicine, the American Pain Society, and the American Society of Addiction Medicine jointly issued the following definition:

> Addiction is a primary, chronic, neurobiological disease, with genetic, psychosocial, and environmental factors influencing its development and manifestations. It is characterized by behaviors that include one or more of the following: impaired control over drug use, compulsive use, continued use despite harm, and craving.

Their definition, went on to say, physical dependence

is a state of being that is manifested by a drug class specific withdrawal syndrome that can be produced by abrupt cessation, rapid dose reduction, decreasing blood level of the drug, and/or administration of an antagonist. Tolerance is the body's physical adaptation to a drug: greater amounts of the drug are required over time to achieve the initial effect as the body . . . adapts to the intake.

The *Diagnostic and Statistical Manual of Mental Disorders* doesn't use the word *addiction* at all. Instead it has a section about substance dependence:

When an individual persists in use of alcohol or other drugs despite problems related to use of the substance, substance dependence may be diagnosed. Compulsive and repetitive use may result in tolerance to the effect of the drug and withdrawal symptoms when use is reduced or stopped. This, along with Substance Abuse, are considered Substance Use Disorders.

The National Institute on Drug Abuse suggests the following definition:

Addiction is a complex but treatable condition. It is characterized by compulsive drug craving, seeking, and use that persist even in the face of severe adverse consequences. For most people, addiction becomes chronic, with relapses possible even after long periods of abstinence. As a chronic, recurring illness, addiction may require continued treatments to increase the intervals between relapses and diminish their intensity. Through treatment tailored to individual needs, people with drug addiction can recover and lead fulfilling lives.

In 2011, the American Society of Addiction Medicine (ASAM) released a new definition of addiction highlighting that addiction is a chronic brain disorder and not simply a behavioral problem involving too much alcohol, drugs, gambling, or sex. (The ASAM provides the public and medical professionals with valuable information, guidance, and research on addiction.) This was the first time the ASAM took an official position that addiction is not solely related to problematic substance use. Here is a somewhat shortened version of their most recent definition of addiction:

Addiction is a primary, chronic disease of brain reward, motivation, memory and related circuitry. Dysfunction in these circuits leads to characteristic biological, psychological, social and spiritual manifestations. This is reflected in an individual pathologically pursuing reward and/or relief by substance use and other behaviors.

"At its core, addiction isn't just a social problem or a moral problem or a criminal problem. It's a brain problem whose behaviors manifest in all these other areas," said

Michael Miller, the past president of the ASAM who oversaw the development of the new definition. "Many behaviors driven by addiction are real problems and sometimes criminal acts. But the disease is about brains, not drugs. It's about underlying neurology, not outward actions."

The landmark study by Columbia University's Center on Addiction and Substance Abuse, published in 2014, refined the definition further: "Addiction is a complex disease, often chronic in nature, which affects the structure and function of the brain. It can be effectively prevented, treated and managed by medical and other health professionals."

Why do the words used to describe addiction matter? People use many words interchangeably when talking about addiction, including *experimentation, use, misuse, hazardous use, excessive use, risky behavior, abuse,* and *dependence.* If those of us who treat addiction cannot agree on the exact wording of a definition—or even if we should use the word *addiction* at all—it is difficult to engender confidence among the general public.

People need things well defined and perfectly clear in order to make informed decisions regarding their health and the well-being of family members. Unless we can agree on standardized terms, the ability to properly diagnose the chronic disease of addiction is jeopardized.

Chapter 4

The Medical Consequences of Addiction

Americans have a curious, inconsistent perspective on alcohol and drug addiction. Studies have shown that the majority of Americans now believe that genetics and biological factors play a role in the development of addiction. However, when asked about it in a different way, a recent survey revealed only 34 percent of American adults saw addiction as primarily a disease or a health problem.

It's tempting to blame an ill-informed public on this apparent contradiction, but even 43 percent of the physicians when polled said that alcoholism is primarily the result of a personal weakness or moral failing. But as a physician for five years in the ER at Los Angeles County General Hospital, treating the physical effects of lives ravaged by alcohol and drugs on a daily basis, I know that addiction is a serious disease that requires medical care.

Addiction contributes to more than seventy other conditions requiring medical attention. While each popular addictive drug differs in its effect on the body, there are overlapping medical consequences, including brain damage, psychiatric symptoms and syndromes (delusion, paranoia, anxiety, and depression), and physical symptoms from gastrointestinal (extreme stomachaches, terrible pain, and uncontrollable diarrhea and vomiting) to increased risk of hypertension, high blood pressure, heart disease, liver disease, various cancers, bone fractures, pancreatitis, pneumonia, hepatitis, kidney failure, ulcers, and urinary tract infections.

For women, addiction can result in the end of menstruation, miscarriages, and children with birth defects (more on the needless tragedy of fetal alcohol syndrome in Chapter 10). For men, addiction can result in shrunken testicles and impotency. But perhaps the most sobering statistics concerning the medical consequences of addiction is the heightened occurrence of suicide: Approximately 18 percent of alcoholics commit suicide and more than 50 percent of all suicides are associated with alcohol or drug dependence.

Neurological Impairment

All excessive behaviors have consequences. If people drink too much alcohol, they first lose coordination, and then their thinking gets screwed up. This is called *neurological impairment*. It is also called being really drunk.

Despite alcohol consumption being both socially acceptable and perfectly legal, it inflicts more damage and kills more people than any other drug in the United States. Alcohol is the third leading cause of death because it attacks every vital organ system in the human body. Simply put, the list of medical problems directly related to immoderate use of alcohol is more than all other recreational drugs combined.

Alcohol may mix harmlessly in polite social settings where moderation and decorum are the established and observed standards, but alcoholism is something else entirely. Those who overindulge in alcohol often use other drugs as well, and that's a big problem. Alcohol does not mix well with anything else. For example, there is a potentially dangerous interaction between cocaine and alcohol. This mixture is the most common two-drug combination that results in drug-related death. Also, mixing alcohol and heroin may be the true reason for overdose deaths attributed to heroin.

I previously mentioned the various types of damage alcohol can do to your body. If you want a more detailed list of alcohol-related damage, here it is: high blood pressure, damage to the heart muscle, heart failure, strokes, severe thiamine deficiency, diabetes, pancreatitis, night blindness, pneumonia, dehydration, kidney failure, vitamin D deficiency leading to bone fractures, inflammation of the digestive system, ulcers, holes in the intestines or stomach, infections of the urinary tract, and, ultimately, death from alcohol poisoning, excessive intoxication, and organ malfunction.

I haven't even mentioned sexual problems (such as erectile dysfunction and impotence), cirrhosis of the liver, and long-term brain damage. Your liver can handle only one drink per hour.

Binge drinking is devastating to the liver. Between 10 and 35 percent of alcoholics have hepatitis or inflamed livers. Cirrhosis occurs when healthy liver cells become replaced by scar tissue. The damage can be so bad that the only treatment option is a liver transplant.

Alcohol slows your reactions, impairs your decision-making abilities, and makes performance of any task requiring accuracy pretty much a lost cause. Alcohol increases confidence but reduces performance. You do everything worse on alcohol, and everyone knows it except the person on alcohol.

Drinking alcohol in extreme weather conditions can be suicidal. Drinking to warm up in the freezing cold has the exact opposite effect. You think you are warmer because of increased blood flow at the surface of your skin, but you are actually losing heat quicker.

If you keep drinking when you have cirrhosis of the liver, you will most likely be dead within seven years. In the meantime, you can develop kidney failure and all kinds of disturbing brain disorders.

Brain Damage

Damage to the brain first shows up as headaches, blackouts, and numbness in the hands and feet. Keep on drinking and you can have permanent structural damage and premature aging. A thirty-five-year-old alcoholic may well have the shriveled up brain of a sick seventy-year-old.

You can tell when this brain destruction is going on. Between

45 and 70 percent of alcoholics do not perform well on tests of problem solving, abstract thinking, memory, and shifting concepts. About 10 percent have serious impairments.

As long as we're talking about brain damage, let's not ignore impairment to the entire central nervous system, which causes alcoholic blackouts, memory loss, seizures, convulsions, delusions, hallucinations, dementia, and violent behavior.

Psychiatric Problems

More than 40 percent of investigated alcoholics turn out to have one or more psychiatric conditions. Research also shows that out of the group of people with a psychiatric disorder, 28 percent suffer from alcohol dependence. So the question often asked is, What came first, the psychological problem or the alcohol problem?

Yes.

Alcohol and other drug use can *cause* psychiatric symptoms and *mimic* psychiatric syndromes. Alcohol can cause delusion, auditory and visual hallucinations, anxiety, and depression. Some patients may experience auditory hallucinations for weeks or months after they stop drinking and are then misdiagnosed as schizophrenic.

According to a recent study, people with alcohol problems have psychiatric disorders almost twice as often as those who don't have alcohol problems. Drinking and drugging can initiate psychiatric disorders and make them worse. It can also *mask* psychiatric symptoms. Withdrawal can cause psychiatric symptoms and mimic symptoms.

It is also very possible for psychiatric disorders and alcohol and drug problems to exist independently of each other.

To make it even more complicated, psychiatric behaviors can be misinterpreted as drug and alcohol problems. This is one more strong argument for diagnosis by an addiction medicine specialist before initiating treatment as well as for a psychiatric evaluation.

Suicide in a Bottle

There is a high rate of suicide in chronic alcoholics, which increases the longer a person drinks. Approximately 18 percent of alcoholics commit suicide, and more than 50 percent of all suicides are associated with alcohol or drug dependence.

Because alcohol is not digested but absorbed directly through the lining of your mouth, throat, stomach, and intestines, it irritates these organs' linings. The result: gastrointestinal disease accompanied by horrid stomachaches, terrible pain, and uncontrollable diarrhea.

If alcoholics didn't already have enough problems, add being undernourished. That doesn't sound so bad until you realize it means your pancreas isn't going to work right. That makes more work for your liver. Your glucose levels are low, and that causes more brain damage.

If you're a guy, and you want shriveled, shrunken testicles and a nice set of man boobs, keep drinking. Your testosterone levels drop with excessive alcohol use, as does your sperm count. You won't have to worry about sex issues, because you will probably be impotent and unable to have sex anyway.

Female alcoholics often quit menstruating, begin early menopause, or menstruate without ovulation. If they get pregnant, they often miscarry. The babies who survive often suffer from fetal alcohol syndrome.

Other Addictive Substances

Although alcohol is the most destructive and dangerous of all social and recreational intoxicants, there are medical dangers in the misuse of even a benign medication.

OPIOIDS

Pain is one of the most common reasons people consult a physician. The most effective pain relief is from opioid analgesics—narcotic painkillers.

Medications that fall within this class include hydrocodone (for example, Vicodin), oxycodone (OxyContin, Percocet), morphine (Kadian, Avinza), and codeine. Heroin, which was once prescribed as a painkiller, is the most widely used illicit opioid.

You may become physically dependent on painkillers if you take them regularly, but physical dependence is not the disease of addiction. If you stop taking them abruptly, you may develop nausea, sweating, chills, diarrhea, and shaking. When people take these medications for pleasure instead of pain reduction, there is a heightened risk of the disease of addiction.

The FDA estimates that more than 33 million Americans aged twelve and older misused extended-release and long-acting opioids during 2007—up from 29 million just five years earlier. And in 2006, nearly 50,000 emergency room visits were related to opioids.

According to former FDA commissioner Margaret A. Hamburg, "Opioid drugs have benefit when used properly and are a necessary component of pain management for certain patients, but we know that they pose serious risks when used improperly— with serious negative consequences for individuals, families, and communities."

Heroin was synonymous with rock-n-roll, and heroin overdoses were involved in the deaths of such musical luminaries as Tim Buckley, Kurt Cobain, Janis Joplin, Jim Morrison, and Sid Vicious. Like any street drug, heroin is dangerous by virtue of the fact that it is not regulated. If anything, the drug is more dangerous than at the height of the hippie drug culture of the 1960s and 1970s. Joplin likely overdosed on heroin that was 3 to 5 percent pure. Today's ultrapure smack can be 95 percent heroin. There's no evidence that actor Philip Seymour Hoffman's death by heroin overdose in 2014 was related to a suicide. It was ruled accidental in that he simply took too high of a dose of heroin.

However, contrary to public opinion, taking multiple regulated prescription painkillers in relatively low doses does not safeguard the user. Like Hoffman, Oscar-nominated actor Heath Ledger died of an opioid overdose, but the poison of his choice was a dizzying array of prescription pills. His autopsy showed that he didn't die from a large dose of any one drug (like Hoffman's overdose of heroin) but rather the cumulative effect of simultaneous and relative small doses of oxycodone, hydrocodone, alprazolam, diazepam, temazepam, and doxylamine. Taken together, they proved to be a fatal drug cocktail.

STIMULANTS

Cocaine is a stimulant, as is caffeine. Obviously, cocaine is stronger. Amphetamines are also stimulants and have proper medical uses. Methamphetamine, stronger yet, also is used medicinally. Recent studies show promise in using methamphetamine in the treatment of various conditions, including Alzheimer's disease. Amphetamines are prescribed appropriately and safely for children as young as six years of age without ill effect. As with all medicines, appropriate use for a specific condition is beneficial. Misuse and abuse, however, cause all manner of problems.

When stimulants are taken in excess for recreation, the consequences can be delusions, anxiety, hypertension, seizures, stroke, arrhythmia, chest pain, heart attack, and hyperthermia. Long-term meth misuse can cause extreme psychosis similar to schizophrenia.

There's the misguided idea that cocaine addiction is somehow easier to control than other drugs. It's not. The deaths of John Belushi, Whitney Houston, and Robin Williams are all associated directly or indirectly with the drug.

Cocaine abuse is also associated with numerous detrimental health effects. Ten cocaine-induced psychiatric disorders are described in the *Diagnostic and Statistical Manual of Mental Disorders*, all of them the result of continued excessive indulgence.

COKE BUGS

Coke bugs, meth mites, and speed bugs are common names used for the delusion that there are bugs crawling on your skin, under your skin, or infesting your clothing, furniture, or even your pets. Amphetamines, methamphetamine, and/or cocaine can cause the physical sensation known as *formication*, which, when combined with the seeking, searching, and exploring behavior that is symptomatic of stimulant overuse, gives rise to the false belief of infestation and parasitic insect activity. The obsession over or observation of nonexistent bugs is called *parasitosis*.

With cocaine and methamphetamine, this phenomenon occurs because the human body can't digest the hazardous additives, or "cut," that were mixed in to increase the seller's profit margin. The body forces these toxic substances out through the pores, causing sores, acne, and chronic scratching.

Stimulants also cause your body temperature to go up, and you begin to perspire heavily. When the sweat evaporates, it removes the skin's protective oils. The combined effects of sweating, lack of protective oils, and dehydration creates a sensation that feels like something irritating or crawling on or under the skin (delusional parasitosis).

This phenomenon was first noted in the 1890s and has been observed in all decades subsequently. In addition, people suffering from stimulant overuse find their attention directed to raised follicles or small irregularities in the skin, and they pick or pluck at these until they have numerous scars and lesions.

Extreme use of stimulants and the subsequent lack of sleep

and nutrition may result in someone spending hours searching through his clothes or bedding with a magnifying glass for evidence of bugs. Some resort to microscopes in their quest, and it is common for those suffering from this delusion to bring evidence to doctors, pest controllers, or skin specialists. Believing they have captured one or more of these bugs, they are often upset when a doctor informs them that their evidence is nothing more than a piece of their own skin, a remnant of a scab, or a piece of lint.

In more advanced stages of this delusion, people cut their skin open to find the bugs or pluck all the hair follicles out of various areas of their body. I had one female patient who was convinced that not only she had these bugs but her dog had them too. The innocent creature was subjected to hour on hour of her plucking away at it with tweezers until the poor thing was virtually hairless.

PARANOIA

When people are paranoid, they distrust the behavior and motives of others. They view even the most innocent actions with suspicion. Among the drugs that can cause paranoia are corticosteroid medications, H_2 blockers (cimetidine, ranitidine, famotidine), some muscle relaxants (baclofen), antiviral/anti-Parkinson's drugs (amantadine), some amphetamines (methylphenidate, or Ritalin), anti-HIV medications and antidepressants (Nardil). Paranoia can be prompted by the abuse of alcohol, cocaine, marijuana, ecstasy (MDMA), amphetamines (including Ritalin), LSD, and PCP (angel dust).

A common symptom of stimulant overuse is paranoia coupled with hypervigilance. This is known in the drug world as *tweaking*. Affected people actually stand at the door and peer through the peep hole, attempting to see if someone is sneaking up on them or stand and stare out the window blinds as if anticipating an attack.

While this is often described as a negative effect of cocaine or other stimulant use, research shows that some people actually enjoy hypervigilance and paranoid delusions. Stop and think about this for a moment. When you read a list of the ill effects of using stimulants for recreation, one of the bad things is paranoid delusions and fear, along with elevated heart rate. The same could be said for scary movies, and it is precisely to heighten the intensity of these fears that some people indulge in the misuse of these drugs.

"I like being paranoid," confessed one of my patients. "I know that my fear isn't really real any more than the fear from watching a horror movie. I know in the back of my head that this feeling is temporary, like the scary rides at an amusement park. Lots of folks don't like the feeling, but I do. In fact, the scary feeling is the reason I like to get high."

Most people who have paranoid delusions, however, do not find it entertaining, and these delusions can result in violence against people whom the paranoid person imagines as enemies.

MARIJUANA

When alcohol was illegal in the United States, marijuana was the only legal recreational drug available. The roles were soon reversed, and marijuana's reputation went into stark decline for several decades. Today, however, marijuana is the most commonly used drug among teenagers in the United States, and it is destined to become more popular as the legalization movement takes hold in Colorado, Washington, and other states. While alcohol is far and away the most destructive intoxicant, the combination of alcohol and marijuana is especially harmful to the developing brains of adolescents.

The human brain develops up to 400 percent more receptors for the active ingredients in marijuana if use begins in the early teenage years, and consistent use during this critical period may give rise to various neurological and psychological issues, including problems with verbal skills, sequential memory processing, motivation, and task completion.

Frequent adolescent marijuana users manifest significant impairments to important cognitive brain functions, and the negative effect of marijuana on memory and concentration is well documented. Those who begin marijuana use at the age when the brain is still developing may be more vulnerable to various neurological and psychological issues, including problems with their verbal skills.

Marijuana smokers also have a lower rate of college acceptance and a higher dropout rate, although poor academic performance often comes before the marijuana use and is one of the triggers for the onset of drug use. Once started, however, the usage combines with collateral sociological and emotional factors to further undermine the student's academic career. While it is true that there are pot smokers at Harvard and Yale, these are incredibly bright achievers who were always top academic performers, and they certainly did not spend their adolescence "wasted" instead of studying.

Another result of prolonged use of marijuana is reduced sperm count, verified by a study conducted by the American Society for Reproductive Medicine. "The bottom line is, the active ingredients in marijuana are doing something to sperm, and the numbers are in the direction toward infertility," said Lani J. Burkman, lead author on the study. "The sperm from marijuana smokers were moving too fast too early," she added. "The timing was all wrong. These sperm will experience burnout before they reach the egg and would not be capable of fertilization."

As an addiction specialist, I've treated patients with marijuana withdrawal symptoms of anxiety, agitation, insomnia, and even violent behavior. These patients struggle to stay away from marijuana with the same challenges as those who have battles with alcohol or other drugs, and their psychological pain is obviously visible and confirmed by the patients themselves.

MEDICAL MARIJUANA

In my opinion, medical marijuana continues to make a mockery of medicine. Let me begin with the fact that the approval process is outright laughable. Anyone with a checkbook can get a recommendation letter for marijuana.

Under normal standards of professional care, a doctor performs a complete physical examination and diagnosis of the patient and then prescribes appropriate medication. Once the medical treatment begins, there is continual interaction between doctor and patient to ascertain the progress and efficacy of the treatment.

In the case of medical marijuana, there is no standard medical procedure performed, no special training for the physicians, and no guidelines. There is also no prescription written, nor are there any specifics as to dose and frequency. You can get a marijuana card for as little as $35 if your complaint is "hair pain" or something equally dubious.

Anyone with any symptom can go to a marijuana doctor and can get a recommendation letter stating that the person will medically benefit from marijuana. The patient then takes this letter to a marijuana dispensary and picks out the flavor of marijuana he or she finds most appealing.

This isn't a prescription such as "take 500 milligrams 3 times a day for 30 days," and no one in the dispensary, including the patient, has any idea what it is he or she is getting.

Marijuana in a Pill

Medical marijuana in pill form, sold under the brand name Marinol, is a legal prescription medication used to treat the adverse effects of chemotherapy and to increase appetite in AIDS patients. The active ingredient is synthetic THC, and Marinol is approved by the medical community and the FDA, the nation's watchdog over unsafe and harmful food and drug products.

Why not just smoke it? Smoking is generally a poor way to deliver medicine. As a doctor, I assure you that it is almost impossible to administer safe, regulated dosages of medicines in smoked form. Morphine, for example, has proven to be a medically valuable drug, but no responsible physician endorses smoking opium or heroin.

Another reason for not smoking marijuana for its medical properties is the issue of tar. While tar is one of the most dangerous aspects of smoking tobacco, the tar level in marijuana is 400 percent higher than in tobacco. Of course, even heavy pot smokers do not smoke pot at the same level that tobacco smokers smoke cigarettes. If they did, they would have far more problems to worry about than tar.

There are profound reasons for addiction medicine specialists, as well as other physicians, to look askance at the current so-called medical marijuana programs in California as well as in other states.

Rather than further disgrace the medical profession with absurd claims of medical marijuana, it would make more sense to legalize marijuana as a recreational intoxicant, tax it, and use the revenue for public education and medical rehabilitation of those who have suffered marijuana's negative consequences.

Just as the vast majority of people who drink are neither problem drinkers nor alcoholics, the majority of adults who smoke marijuana are not problem smokers or drug addicts. My concerns are in two categories.

First, because marijuana is illegal, there are no regulatory standards of production and manufacture regarding content and potency. Hence, one cannot state that marijuana used properly is safe because there is no definition of *properly* nor is there a standard safe dosage. Second, there is a predictable percentage of people who, due to genetics and other factors, will manifest the disease of addiction. One out of six people who smoke marijuana regularly develop problems requiring some type of medical intervention.

Like all other mind-altering drugs, marijuana is definitely dangerous in combination with any motor vehicle. It affects alertness, concentration, coordination, and reaction time. Marijuana also makes it hard to judge distances. The worst-case scenario is combining marijuana with even a small amount of alcohol. The two together are more dangerous on the road than either drug alone.

BARBITURATES AND TRANQUILIZERS

Barbiturates were first used in medicine in the early 1900s and became popular in the 1960s and 1970s for treatment of anxiety, insomnia, and seizure disorders. They evolved into recreational drugs that some people used to reduce inhibitions, decrease anxiety, and to treat unwanted side effects of other illicit drugs.

Barbiturate use and abuse has declined dramatically since the 1970s, mainly because a safer group of sedative-hypnotics called benzodiazepines is being prescribed. In the day, barbiturates abuse caused, or was significantly involved, in many of the most high-profile overdose deaths in the entertainment industry including those of Judy Garland (1969), Jimi Hendrix (1970), and Elvis Presley (1977).

Medications such as Valium and Xanax are some of the most commonly prescribed benzodiazepine medications, also known as tranquilizers, in the United States. There are numerous uses for these medications, but when people take them who don't need them, there are problems. People at risk for addiction to these substances are also at risk for alcoholism. The combination of the two is deadly.

Withdrawal from benzodiazepines is similar to alcohol withdrawal and can be a dangerous process if not done properly. One should never stop these drugs cold turkey but instead taper off the doses, as directed by a physician.

While benzodiazepine was designed as a safer alternative to barbiturates, it too was involved in some high-profile overdose deaths in Hollywood, including those of Michael Jackson (2009) and Anna Nicole Smith (2007).

Social Consequences

The idea that there are social consequences for indulging in recreational drug use has come under intense research and professional scrutiny in recent years. In the United States, the biggest social consequence risk for the nonaddict drug user is arrest and or coerced "treatment" for possession of a controlled substance.

According to the National Institute on Drug Abuse (NIDA), "Among young people in drug abuse treatment, marijuana accounts for the largest percentage of admissions: 61 percent of those under age 15 and 56 percent of those 15–19." According to the U.S. government study from which NIDA gets this figure, the majority of these teens were not in treatment because of dependence or addiction. They were given a choice of treatment or juvenile detention after being caught in possession of marijuana. There was no medical diagnosis of dependence or addiction.

The National Institute on Drug Abuse doesn't mention this fact because, as an official representative of federal drug policy, it wants the reader to infer the admissions are due to dependence and addiction. Sadly, this is exactly the type of thing that causes teens not to trust antidrug pamphlets. Once again, we see research studies used not as education but as propaganda. While the intent may be honorable, the methods undermine credibility and perpetuate harmful exaggerations.

Because of my role as a doctor who treats patients with the medical condition of addiction, you might think I would approve of any method that proposes to decrease drug use. Proposing isn't the same as accomplishing, and falsely labeling people as drug addicts when they do not have the disease of addiction diminishes the credibility of the condition itself and makes a mockery of treatment.

A 2004 conference on special designer drugs and cocaine held in Bern, Switzerland, prominently featured extensive research by Peter Cohen, author of "The Social and Health Consequences of Cocaine Use." In his final analysis, and in his words, "For all drug use and drug users, social exclusion and marginalization are the worst settings. The best harm and crime reduction money can buy is to lower marginalization and exclusion of drug users, even if this would mean that the drugs they (still) like to use have to be made available to them at acceptable costs. In my view, daily and regular use is far less of a danger to people than social exclusion."

We must deal with what is real, and the reality is that I

practice addiction medicine in the United States, where the stigma against addicts is widespread, punitive legal measures are still instituted against disease sufferers, and millions of people who could avoid addiction or be treated successfully receive no help beyond a good scolding, shame, a jail sentence, and marginally helpful support group meetings.

The Criminalization of a Disease

If you thought you had cancer, you would go to a cancer specialist for medical diagnosis. You may also attend a support group for people dealing with cancer, but you would certainly pursue effective medical treatment. It is the same with heart disease, diabetes, and asthma. These are all chronic medical conditions with strong emotional and environmental components. They are all also preventable and treatable. So is addiction.

The difference, however, between addiction and every other chronic disease in the United States is that addiction is criminalized to a large degree. In federal prisons in 2014, 52.1 percent (95,079 of 182,333 prisoners) were there for drug-related crimes. Another 265,000 prisoners are in state prisons on drug charges.

More than 1.6 million people are arrested, prosecuted, and imprisoned each year for a drug law violation. The vast majority of these crimes are nonviolent, yet the violence to society because of these draconian, antiquated drug laws is immense. Nearly $33 billion each year is spent on keeping prisoners behind bars in federal and state prisons for drug-related charges. Of course, this doesn't count the incalculable costs of lives ruined and families destroyed.

I want to stress, it is not a crime in the United States to have the physical illness of addiction. But if the object of your addiction, such as illicit drugs, is illegal, you could be arrested and prosecuted for the mere act of possessing it. The situation places the person suffering from addiction in a situation of continually interacting with the criminal underworld rather than with medical professionals.

Numerous studies show it's much less expensive to treat people with drug problems than to toss them into prison. A 1994 Rand analysis concluded that for every extra dollar spent on addiction treatment, taxpayers save $7.46 in societal expenses, including the cost of incarceration.

The United States has about 5 percent of the world's population, but we have 25 percent of the world's prisoners—we incarcerate a greater percentage of our population than any country on earth. We have earned the unenviable nickname of Incarceration Nation.

An article titled "Medicine and the Epidemic of Incarceration in the United States" published in the *New England Journal of Medicine* reviewed the deplorable plight of drug-addicted and mentally ill inmates in our nation's prisons and concluded:

> *Locking up millions of people for drug-related crimes has failed as a public-safety strategy and has harmed*

public health in the communities to which these men and women return. A new evidence-based approach is desperately needed. We believe that in addition to capitalizing on the public health opportunities that incarceration presents, the medical community and policymakers must advocate for alternatives to imprisonment, drug-policy reform, and increased public awareness of this crisis in order to reduce mass incarceration and its collateral consequence.

Chapter 5

The Process of Effective Treatment

I have a chronic disease called diabetes. There's no cure for my chronic disease, but I maintain a fairly normal and, some would say, highly successful life. How do I do it? I follow a strict regimen of medications formulated to address my particular disease. I also modify my lifestyle to minimize the risks associated with my disease.

Now as a diabetic, not to mention a physician, I would no more think that I could treat my disease by sitting around in a room with other diabetics and commiserating about our problems than thinking I could cure it by eating a diet of only chocolate cake. These are but ridiculous propositions—yet, that is, in effect, the expectation we have for those who suffer from the chronic disease of alcohol and drug addiction.

In western Europe, drug policies differ from country to country but focus first and foremost on providing evidence-based treatment to addicts rather than criminalization of substance abuse. Portugal has decriminalized drug possession in small amounts altogether. Germany, too, focuses on treatment, but still aggressively pursues drug trafficking. While still criminalizing possession, German prosecutors have moved away from pressing charges to emphasizing treatment. The Netherlands, famous for its legalized cannabis bars, nevertheless has taken new steps to crack down on the smuggling of so-called hard drugs, such as opium and heroin. The result of these harm-reduction programs has been a massive decrease in new drugs users, with Portugal decreasing by 38 percent, the Netherlands by 24 percent, and Germany by 17 percent.

The standard for addiction treatment in the United States—unlike all other Western nations—is a program based on a seventy-five-year-old philosophy in which sharing stories is the focus. The organization that offers this philosophy, Alcoholics Anonymous, makes no claims to having helped the majority of people with substance addiction or even the majority of people who come to it for help. By its own estimates, it is probably effective in treating addiction over the long-term for only 5 percent of those who have attended one of their group meetings.

Now, you may say that no one forces anyone to seek help for addiction treatment from AA, but that's not true. For the most part, drug courts in the United States assign mandatory treatment for those convicted of minor drug-related criminal activity (mostly possession of small amounts of illicit drugs) to so-called rehab clinics whose treatment consists mostly or exclusively of AA treatment protocols. That's a fancy way of saying that their patients sit in a room and talk about their drug problems. If they're lucky, the discussion might be led by a drug counselor, but more often than not, it's lead by someone who doesn't even have a college degree much less any medical training and whose only qualification frequently is that they, too, are recovering from an alcohol or drug addiction.

It's incredible, but that is the sorry state in this country of the treatment of alcohol and drug addiction, the third most widespread chronic disease in America.

A recent nationwide study on alcohol and drug addiction by the National Center on Addiction and Substance Abuse at Columbia University concluded, "Unlike other diseases . . . the vast majority of people in need of addiction treatment do not receive anything that approximates evidence-based care." It goes on to say that the consequences of this failure are "profound," resulting in "an enormous array of health and social problems such as accidents, homicides and suicide, child neglect and abuse, family dysfunction and unplanned pregnancies."

Here's the greatest irony: This chronic disease, unlike Alzheimer's, arthritis, or asthma, for example, is largely preventable. We also know how to effectively treat it with evidence-based medicine.

Addiction Treatment in the Twenty-First Century

I mentioned earlier how the U.S. standard of addiction treatment has nothing to do with medicine. In western Europe, Japan, and most other industrialized nations, treatment of alcohol and drug dependency is grounded in science and research. Now, here in the United States, we offer that same kind of treatment, too, but the difference is that evidence-based treatment is not the standard here.

What is evidence-based treatment of addiction? Evidence-based medicine is simply the application of the scientific method into healthcare. It's the standard for the treatment of every chronic disease in America except substance addiction.

There is absolutely no denying that addiction is a chronic medical illness that must be controlled with proper treatment, including medications—just like my disease of diabetes and other complex and chronic medical conditions.

As a psychiatrist specializing in addiction medicine and who has been treating addicts for the last two decades, I can tell you the answer lies in integrating mental health and addiction treatment into a single, comprehensive program designed to meet the individual needs of each specific patient.

Effective, evidence-based treatment of addiction has three parts that work together:

- *Biomedical*, which focuses on improved detoxification regimens, followed by the use of medicines to reduce cravings and manage addiction over a lifetime and, when appropriate, the application of psychiatric medications.
- *Psychological*, which includes addiction counseling, cognitive behavioral treatment psychotherapy, aversion therapy, and behavioral self-control training.
- *Sociocultural*, which uses the community reinforcement approach, family therapy, therapeutic communities, vocational rehabilitation, various motivational techniques, culturally specific interventions, and contingency management.

All three of these modalities have more than one dimension in common, such as social skills training, relapse prevention techniques, self- and mutual-help programs, support groups, and chemical aversion therapy.

Addiction is a chronic medical condition, a brain disorder. Just as hypertension and asthma have biological, psychological, and social components, so do alcoholism and drug addiction. An evidence-based addiction treatment must include all three components.

Equally important, each program must be individualized for each patient. It's not that the current AA/12-step protocol that characterizes treatment at most rehab clinics is inherently bad. It's just incomplete. Fundamentally, it lacks two of three essential components—biomedical and psychological—needed for a successful treatment of the disease of addiction over the short and long term. It also has a one-size-fits-all mentality in which any deviation from its main tenet—abstinence—is considered heresy. In a disease as complex as substance addiction, that simply does not work for most people.

Here's the good news: Just as the diabetic can live a normal life with certain adjustments (monitoring blood sugar levels, regular medicals exams, taking insulin, modifying diet, and so on), so can the recovering alcoholics or addicts can live normal lives with their own life adjustments.

Assessment

Before evidence-based addiction treatment begins, all patients need a full medical and psychiatric diagnosis and evaluation, plus evaluation of their individual psychological and social situation.

As a part of a comprehensive medical evaluation, an EKG and a complete blood chemical analysis should be performed. A blood metabolic panel is a group of chemical tests that measure the amount of vitamins, minerals, cholesterol, protein, blood sugar, electrolytes, and other bodily requirements and functions.

An EEG, CT, MRI, or PET scan may also be conducted before treatment to ascertain the severity of brain structural or functional damage, or other brain-related concerns. After all, alcoholism and substance misuse are diseases of the brain.

From this information, a physician, preferably one trained in addiction medicine, can determine the severity of the patient's addiction. The American Society of Addiction Medicine, a professional society representing more than 3,200 physicians and associated professionals dedicated to increasing access and improving the quality of addiction treatment, defines six dimensions to addiction severity: (1) potential for acute intoxication and/or withdrawal, (2) biomedical conditions and complications, (3) emotional/behavioral conditions or complications, (4) treatment acceptance/resistance, (5) relapse potential, and (6) recovery environment. The goal is to match the patient's needs to the appropriate treatment service by assessing the severity of the addiction as well as verification of the medical diagnosis.

Key to Effective Treatment

There are very few diseases that are purely biological in nature. The causes of most diseases, including alcohol and drug addiction, are multifaceted, with biomedical, psychological, and sociocultural factors. Effective treatment is achieved when all of these factors are integrated into a comprehensive program.

Let's be clear: The effective treatment of substance addiction is highly individualistic, requiring a trained physician to assess both the patient's physical and psychological condition. For some patients, no psychological treatment is required; for others, it becomes a primary focus. Sometimes counseling that includes a patient's family is absolutely necessary (and this is especially true with teen addicts), but in other cases it's not necessary and is even counterproductive. Rehab clinics that offer a standard treatment for all patients are engaging in the worst kind of breach of medical ethics. They either know better or should know better.

Despite the individualistic approach required in effective addiction treatment, this I know for certain: The successful treatment of alcohol and drug addiction *must first* address the biological component and correct the brain's chemistry imbalance in the process.

Let's dig a little deeper into each of three parts of an evidence-based treatment.

BIOMEDICAL THERAPY

If we accept the scientifically proven theory that addiction is a medical condition, then we have to recognize that medications can compensate or even reverse the pathology of the disease. When medications work, no matter what the target illness, they have a relatively quick and dramatic effect.

Of the medications that have proven to treat the disease of

addiction, Suboxone, which is the combination of buprenorphine and naloxone (the drug used by first responders to reverse the effect of an overdose), is the most successful. Suboxone mimics the effects of opioids like heroin, in effect, by occupying the receptors that opioids affect. If someone on Suboxone injects heroin, he feels little effect. And because the medication mimics an opioid, there's little craving. Unlike methadone, which has a similar if not albeit more crude effect, Suboxone doesn't have to be administered via a daily visit to a clinic. Suboxone is a pill of a sublingual (under the tongue) form that can be prescribed to the patient by an authorized doctor.

Several other drugs for treating addictions have been approved in recent years, adding to the portfolio already in use. Clonidine is used for heroin and opiate addiction and naltrexone, acamprosate, gabapentin, and topiramate for alcoholism (we will delve deeper into each of these medications further in the book).

It's important to emphasize again that each individual patient will respond differently to different medications and different dosages. That's why it is essential that biomedical therapy only be administered under the supervision of trained medical professionals.

PSYCHOLOGICAL THERAPY

Most chemically dependent people and those with mental disorders feel overwhelmed and helpless. They yearn for hope and a sense of empowerment in the face of debilitating disease. An important aspect of effective treatment includes empowering patients to see themselves in partnership with their physician, strengthening their physical, emotional, and mental health.

As the disease of addiction impacts the thought processes, another important aspect of effective treatment is individualized cognitive behavioral therapy (CBT). This therapy is a form of psychotherapy that emphasizes the important role of thinking how we feel and what we do.

There are several approaches to cognitive behavioral therapy, including rational emotive behavior therapy, rational behavior therapy, rational living therapy, cognitive therapy, and dialectic behavior therapy. All of these cognitive behavioral therapies are based on the idea that our thoughts cause our feelings and behaviors, not external things like people, situations, or events. Even if a situation remains unchanged, how we respond to that situation can change. We can choose our response, making a conscious decision to respond in ways that are in the best interest of our health and happiness.

In conjunction with CBT, there is another therapy valuable in treating addicts. Motivation enhancement therapy (MET) has been thoroughly researched in the field of substance misuse and has proven to be exceptionally effective at enhancing an individual's motivation to make positive changes in behavior. Also, with many patients, family therapy is also helpful and even essential. Depending on the patient's family dynamic, involving the family in the recovery process can mean the difference between success and failure.

An effective treatment must help patients address, identify, and describe the personal meaning of their addiction. Are they self-medicating, filling up an inner emptiness, numbing feelings related to a trauma, or all of the above? Unless clients understand what they are actually doing on a deep conscious and subconscious level, they will chronically relapse. A responsible, comprehensive treatment program takes all aspects into consideration for the ongoing health and well-being of the patient.

When it works properly, psychological therapy empowers the patient to be her own gatekeeper so she doesn't have to be told (or scolded or shamed) into avoiding behavior that can trigger relapse. Let me give an example.

Motivational Therapy at Work

Maureen was a middle-aged woman who had been referred to me by her primary-care doctor for depression (about 50 percent of all addicts have a mental disorder, and depression is the most common). While interviewing her, it quickly became clear that she had a dual disorder, both clinically depressed and an alcoholic. She drank two to three bottles of wine daily, which was not only making her more depressed but also ruining her physical health. Keep in mind that she had come to visit me only for her depression. Like many addicts, because of their impaired brain function, she didn't think she had a serious addiction.

When I suggested she think about cutting back on her wine because of the grave dangers it was posing to her health, she matter-of-factly stated, "Oh, no. I can't do that. I love my wine." It's as if she were talking about her pet dog. At that moment she could not make the connection between the enormous amounts of alcohol she was consuming and its deleterious effects on her health. Still, I went ahead and prescribed her an antidepressant that would not be dangerous to take with alcohol, nevertheless knowing that the alcohol would negate most of its effect.

Two weeks later when I saw her again, she began the conversation by saying that she had thought about what I had told her about how her large consumption of wine would eventually destroy her health. She said that she was thinking about cutting back. I reinforced her first baby step toward controlling what was obviously a full-blown alcohol addiction by saying that I wanted her to consider decreasing her daily wine consumption by two glasses. I asked if she thought she could manage that, and she affirmed that she could. She also agreed to take a pill called Topamax that helped decrease her cravings for alcohol.

When I saw her next, her depression had begun to ebb (because the medication was at last being given a real chance to work), and she had succeeded in reducing her habit to only six glasses of wine instead of the eight to twelve she had been consuming when she first saw me. I told her that she was doing a great job and that she was ready to take the next step to cut her wine back to only one bottle a day. "You think I can do that?" she asked hesitantly. "Oh, absolutely. As your doctor, I can see you're ready," I told her confidently.

Six months after she first saw me, she achieved complete abstinence from alcohol. Five years later, she is still clean and sober.

Here's what we know in the twenty-first century about the disease of alcohol and drug addiction: Willpower or the lack thereof isn't the cause of the disease. It's the symptom. Successful psychotherapy doesn't shame the patient into abstaining from alcohol or drugs, but rather cultivates that seed of ambivalence within every addict that what she is doing to herself could be very bad for her health. Together, the therapist and patient focus on creating an internally motived change rather than a step-by-step process.

SOCIOCULTURAL THERAPY

According to current brain research and developmental psychology, the risk of addictive disease is heightened by, and directly related to, life experience as much as genetics.

Human are the only species in which the majority of the brain develops after we are born, and what we experience at pivotal points in our life determines a vast amount of our neurological development. For the sake of simplicity, I'll put it this way: You are an individual, and what you experience in your life has just as much impact on your brain functioning as does heredity and genetics.

However, perhaps the most disturbing discovery, repeatedly verified by extensive international research, regarding the disease of addiction is that emotional pain and stress—especially alienation, social exclusion, and emotional distancing—create actual neurological damage that increases the risk of alcoholism and addiction and the risk of never recovering.

Stress has long been known to increase vulnerability to addiction. Research over the last decade has led to a dramatic increase in understanding the underlying mechanisms for this association. Behavioral and neurobiological correlates are being studied and evidence of molecular and cellular changes associated with chronic stress and addiction have been identified.

Effective therapy, then, must identify chronic stress factors in the patient's life and create strategies for resolving them.

Nutrition and exercise also can play important roles in treatment by mitigating the symptoms of detoxification and promoting overall treatment outcomes. Many addicts have unhealthy diets that enhance anxiety. They often turn to sugar and carb-laden junk foods to satisfy their craving because these foods increase serotonin levels. Good nutrition provides a baseline foundation for physical well-being in which all other aspects of treatment from medications to counseling are facilitated.

Exercise can also have a direct effect on maintaining proper neurotransmitter levels in the brain. Because exercise stimulates the dopamine pathways, it can mimic the reward produced by the addict's substance of choice. It also generally helps mitigate the symptoms of depression, from which many addicts suffer. Finally, patients who exercise in groups increase their social skills and create social networks in settings not related directly to their substance abuse.

A New Generation of Addiction Medications

As I mentioned earlier in the text, addiction is a chronic disease characterized by the inability to consistently abstain, by impairment in behavioral control, by cravings, by diminished recognition of significant problems with one's behaviors and interpersonal relationships, and by a dysfunctional emotional response. Like other chronic diseases, addiction often involves cycles of relapse and remission. Without treatment or engagement in recovery activities, addiction is progressive and can result in disability or premature death.

The new generation of addiction medications, which are easy for the patient to take and easy for the physician to administer, are important for two reasons. First, recovery from addiction is hard, and patients need every tool that medicine can offer them. But there is another potential benefit: The growing availability of medical treatments will encourage doctors to treat their patients' addiction problems just as they would a patient's out-of-control blood sugar or high cholesterol.

Second, the emergence of long-acting drugs goes beyond diminishing the pain of detox and actually reduces cravings that persist, even in people who are highly committed to abstinence. Addicts no longer have to summon their willpower alone to take their medications each day. As an added benefit, long-acting drugs reduce the temptation to sell drugs on the street, easing their burden in the challenging first months of recovery.

New, even longer-lasting versions of these drugs will soon be coming to market. For example, Titan Pharmaceuticals is in the process of seeking Food and Drug Administration (FDA) approval of an implant that would provide continuous delivery of the drug buprenorphine—sold as Suboxone in its pill form—for six months to people attempting recovery from dependence on heroin or prescription painkillers. Studies at the University of California, Los

Angeles found that nearly 66 percent of patients who had the implant inserted under the skin in the upper arm stuck with treatment—compared with only 31 percent of those who received a placebo implant. They had higher rates of clean urine tests and lower rates of withdrawal symptoms and cravings.

The National Institute on Drug Abuse is also putting considerable effort into developing vaccines to fight addiction to cocaine, heroin, and methamphetamine. The aim is to trigger an immune response to a drug of abuse so it can't reach the brain and elicit a high, causing cravings for the drug to erode over time.

Treating the Unique Addict or Alcoholic

All addicts and alcoholics think they are unique. In a very true medical sense, they are absolutely correct. No two are the same, and each must receive a thorough medical evaluation to receive the appropriate medical care in a compressive program incorporating all the therapeutic and/or curative methodologies available.

It is interesting that people with a history of drug misuse can take prescription medications that have great potential for abuse and not misuse them. I usually avoid prescribing mood-altering medications, because they may trigger relapse. For selected patients, however, it is both prudent and necessary to use benzodiazepines, such as for patients who are severely bipolar. I also treat patients who have uncontrolled anxiety with other psychiatric medications.

We usually avoid giving patients stimulants unless it turns out that they have undiagnosed attention deficit disorder (ADD). In the majority of those cases, once they are prescribed the most effective stimulant, their life is changed, and their drug misuse ends. For some diagnosed ADD patients who have a nonmedical stimulant dependence, even prescription stimulants trigger a relapse.

Physicians need to keep open minds and provide individualized treatment. The old belief that all addicts are the same is completely wrong. No two are exactly alike, and there is no one treatment that is appropriate for all patients.

To overlook the individuality of the patient is, quite frankly, a gross violation of both ethics and professional responsibility.

Variations in Intoxicated Behavior

ANGER

It is a fact that different people act differently when intoxicated. People often ask me why some people become rude and abusive, even violent, under the influence of alcohol.

The reasons for emotional rage, especially when under the influence, are complex. Comprehensive research regarding anger found that there are medical underpinnings to compulsive, repetitive outbursts of anger, even when not accompanied by ingestion of alcohol, and when the brain imagery of those afflicted indicates the physical disease of addiction along with other medical illnesses.

Researchers at Ohio State University found that men and women with higher levels of hostility also showed higher levels of homocysteine—a blood chemical strongly associated with coronary heart disease. It is medically correct to say that extreme and repetitive anger can cause heart attacks and strokes. There is an ongoing discussion and considerable research concerning hostility and anger because they may be three things at once: a symptom of disease, the cause of disease, or in cases of compulsive rage, a medical condition of an addictive nature.

Jill Bolte Taylor, a trained and published neuroanatomist, garnered acclaim for her specialized postmortem investigation of the human brain as it relates to schizophrenia and severe mental illnesses. According to Taylor, all emotions, including anger, have a chemical component. Once triggered, the brain releases the neurotransmitter dimethyltryptamine (DMT), and you experience the corresponding emotion. Taylor insists that the chemical associated with anger is completely dissipated from the bloodstream in ninety seconds. She asserts that if your anger lasts longer than ninety seconds, it may be that you are self-perpetuating or self-triggering the chemical for much the same reason as a heavy drinker keeps ingesting alcohol.

As a specialist in addiction medicine, I see individuals come to me with highly complex problems involving more than one diagnosis. They may have heart and liver problems, brain dysfunction, addiction, or ulcers plus psychiatric and psychological problems. They may also have any manner of ailments engendered by, aggravated by, or marginally correlated to their compulsive use of alcohol and/or drugs.

Because of both complexity and individuality, there is no simple answer to the question regarding why we have "the angry drunk." There are, however, some interesting recent insights into the phenomenon.

In an experiment at the University of Waterloo in Ontario, Canada, volunteers pressed a particular button when prompted by a computer. These same volunteers were also instructed not to press the button if there was a bright red light. Some participants, when given alcohol, would become defiant. Despite the bright red light, they would smack the button with outright aggression. This is similar to the drunk who does something despite being repeatedly told not to do it.

Furthermore, many studies in the United States have found that a percentage of people who are told they are drinking alcohol behave as if they were under the influence, even becoming aggressive, hostile, and easily sexually aroused—despite not having any alcohol whatsoever.

The reason I introduced those two studies back to back is to raise the obvious question: Is the aggressive and defiant behavior the result of alcohol (or the result of what people believe about the effects of alcohol) or does it indicate another, more subtle medical condition? There is no absolutely correct answer under all circumstances, but we do know that in cultures where alcohol consumption is not associated in any way with aggressive or hostile behavior, the behavior of those who drink is not hostile and aggressive.

The Bad Drunk

The appearance of hostility when drinking is a manifestation of a physical disorder other than alcoholism, even if alcohol addiction is also present. A person who becomes insulting, aggressive, hostile, and/or abusive when drinking, even if he or she rarely touches alcohol, is exhibiting a known symptom of one or more medical conditions other than alcoholism, all of which require comprehensive care by a trained physician. In popular culture, we know this kind of person as a "bad drunk."

The implication for successful treatment of the angry alcoholic is clear: More than the physical illness of addiction must be addressed. There will be more than one diagnosis, and personalized treatment is of paramount importance. As with the alcoholic, solemn oaths to use willpower, the use of support groups, counseling, and the best intentions are, for the most part, useless. Yet, without fail and despite repeated failure, addicts continue to do more of what doesn't work.

Symptoms indicate illness, but symptoms don't diagnose the illness any more than the existence of clues is the answer to a mystery. One symptom or characteristic of addiction is self-stimulation. If an alcoholic has one drink, it stimulates a biochemical and emotional chain reaction triggering the compulsion to keep drinking, despite any unpleasant outcomes. As alcoholism is a medical problem with a biological component of approximately 50 percent, to ignore the physical illness would be irresponsible. Hence simply not drinking is not a medical treatment, although it certainly is a beneficial change in behavior.

If someone is going to assert that anger itself is an addiction or that there are adrenaline addicts, then the people so afflicted should certainly seek the help of a specialist in addiction medicine. Much to my personal shock and dismay, I have seen so-called anger addiction treatments that encourage the "patient" to become angry, express anger, and "get it all out."

When treating alcoholics, it is unlikely that having them drink to excess would be beneficial. I doubt you would buy the alcoholic a case of beer, a large bottle of Scotch, and several wine coolers, and then have him drink to get it out of his system. No responsible person involved in the treatment of addiction would tell drug addicts or alcoholics that they need to drink or drug as much as possible as a way to achieve health and sobriety.

Telling someone with a negative and destructive behavioral addiction not only to continue but also to amplify that behavior, strikes me as both absurd and negligent. After all, with any addiction, the continuation of the behavior ignites a self-stimulating, self-perpetuating system. The more you do, the more you want, even if every indulgence in the addiction brings more pain.

COMPULSION

When compulsion replaces control, the disease of addiction has taken over. There are short episodes of abstinence as a result of coercion or feelings of guilt, shame, or remorse. Those same emotions, however, provide the stress that triggers relapse into active addiction. Once the compulsion is triggered, all efforts at control disintegrate.

When you have an addiction, you look for opportunities to feed your addiction. When the addiction is to alcohol or other drugs, seeking and procuring the drug is part of the obsession; use of the substance is the compulsion.

With an internally stimulated and self-perpetuating brain chemistry, all the addict with compulsive anger issues requires is an insult, real or imagined, to instigate rage. A medical diagnosis, however, would reveal a significant biological factor to the rage issue, in addition to medical problems engendered by the anger itself.

OBSESSION

Obsession is when you can think of only one thing at a time, and it is the same one thing *all* the time. Obsession is an irresistible force of thought that pushes everything else aside.

Obsession is followed by consummation in an unending repetition. For example, stalkers are obsessed with their prey. Fanatics are obsessed by their passions. Active addicts are obsessed with living their addiction.

One psychological attraction of addiction for the intelligent and well informed is the delightful prospect of not being in control. These are people who, due to their important positions of responsibility in life, wish to take a vacation from being in charge and place themselves in a subservient position. Of course, as with the person who pays to visit a dominatrix, they are only pretending not to be in control. In truth, they are in charge of the entire scenario. Sadly, when true addiction manifests itself, the game of "playing a drug addict" is no longer a diversionary vacation but a tragic health crisis.

Addiction is a primary, chronic disease of brain reward, motivation, memory, and related circuitry. Dysfunction in these circuits leads to characteristic biological, psychological, social, and spiritual manifestations. These are reflected in a person's pathological pursuit of reward and/or relief through substance use and other behaviors.

The transition from casual substance use to addiction can be seen in changes in the chemical substances found in the brain, known as neurotransmitters, which transmit messages within the brain's reward system.

Special Considerations for the Opiate Addict

Suboxone, a once-a-day prescription tablet that can be administered only by a physician is a partial opiate, meaning that it gives the brain something similar to what it is used to, without the dangers associated with full opiates. Suboxone contains a combination of two ingredients: buprenorphine and naloxone. Buprenorphine is an opioid medication similar to other opioids, such as morphine, codeine, and heroin.

However, Suboxone doesn't produce the high of those drugs and is therefore easier to stop taking. This has advantages over methadone, although some patients with an exceptionally high degree of addiction are often better candidates for methadone, a medication that has been used effectively and safely to treat opioid addiction for more than thirty years.

HEROIN TREATMENT AND HARM REDUCTION

The heroin that is sold on the streets today is so potent that many patients can't stay away from it, even when under treatment with Suboxone or methadone. This is why nations that adopt a true harm-reduction model of treatment, such as Switzerland, have authorized managed maintenance using actual heroin, medically supervised and dispensed. This reduces both medical harm and social harm by reducing crime and illness.

As we do not yet have this harm-reduction model in the United States, Suboxone is rapidly becoming the medication of choice for managed maintenance for the majority of heroin addicts.

Another advantage of Suboxone is that there is no tolerance developed, but there is a ceiling on the drug's effect. In other words, if you take more than your required amount, you won't get more high.

For extreme opiate-dependent patients, the managed use of Suboxone makes it possible for them to acquire the life skills and personal balance to ride out their addiction without crashing. When they have internalized and integrated the therapeutic tools given to them, these patients recognize the right time to taper off the use of Suboxone until it is completely discontinued.

Remember, we are dealing with a physical disease that can be treated in much the same manner as we treat heart disease, diabetes, or high blood pressure. Whether a patient should take medication for his or her condition, what medication would be most effective, and how long that medication should be administered are matters best determined by the treating physician in consultation with the individual patient.

The Measure of Success

In 1964, the World Health Organization noted, "There is scarcely any agent which can be taken into the body to which some individuals will not get a reaction satisfactory or pleasurable to them,

persuading them to continue its use even to the point of abuse—
that is, to excessive or persistent use beyond medical need."

More than half a century later, that pronouncement rings
truer than ever. The speed at which new drugs surface to join the
already copious ranks of evergreen substances like alcohol, heroin, marijuana, meth, morphine, and prescription painkillers is
amazing. As I write this, the latest trending street drug is something called Flakka, a synthetic drug that produces violent, hallu-
cinatory behavior. It replaces last year's trending drug that
produces violent hallucinations, bath salts.

According to *Forbes* magazine, Flakka is imported from China
or Pakistan and is either smoked, snorted, or injected. It "induces
rapid body-temperature elevation, the need to disrobe and a psychotic
paranoia convincing the user that he is being chased. It can raise
body temperature up to 106 degrees, and like amphetamines, it creates a state of excited delirium." It's even nicknamed $5 insanity.

Why would anyone take such a drug? Of course, there is no
answer to that question.

In the field of drugs, if you build it, they will try it. And that's
the point I'm making. We'll never stop the ingestion of addictive
substances. We as a species lost that battle when we made the
first wine about 6000 B.C.E.

Our society must switch the focus from trying to stop people
from drugging and drinking (remember how well forced abstinence during Prohibition turned out) to providing effective,
evidence-based treatment.

Yes, but how can we possibly know when we've achieved
effective treatment?

The measure of the success of the outcome of treatment is

really quite simple: Does treatment improve the quality of life of the patient? Addiction treatment is successful if the patient can lead a fulfilling, productive, and relatively normal life. It's as simple as that because that is the measure for any medical condition for which there is no cure.

The Modern-Day Medicine Chest for Addiction Treatment

Like other leading chronic diseases, addiction can be controlled and managed with a combination of medication, psychological counseling, and lifestyle choices, so that the addict can experience a fulfilling life.

A number of medications work on the brain circuitry to decrease cravings and, in some instances, the physical symptoms from addiction withdrawal. A short list follows, categorized by addictive substance. Brand names of the medications appear in parentheses.

A physician trained in addiction medicine knows best how to combine these medications in a way that optimizes treatment for each individual patient.

ALCOHOL

- *Acamprosate* (Campral): reduces cravings for alcohol, normalizes brain function affected by heavy alcohol consumption.

- *Baclofen* (Kemstro, Lioresal, Gablofen): reduces cravings and withdrawal symptoms.

- *Disulfiram* (Antabuse): most commonly used aversion medication for alcohol abuse.

- *Naltrexone* (Revia): reduces the high associated with substance or alcohol use, administered as a daily pill (Revia) or monthly injection (Vivitrol), both FDA approved.

- *Ondansetron* (Zofran): antinausea drug shown to be effective in decreasing alcohol cravings, especially effective in those with early-onset addiction.

- *Topiramate* (Topamax): anticonvulsant that may reduce the release of dopamine, thus reducing the rewarding effects of alcohol.

MARIJUANA

- *Gabapentin* (Fanatrex, Gabarone, Gralise, Neurontin): drug for epileptic seizures but also effective in reducing withdrawal symptoms from heavy marijuana users.

- *N-acetylcysteine*: shown to be effective in decreasing cravings for marijuana.

- *Oral tetrahydrocannabinol* (THC) made from psychoactive ingredient in cannabis, shown to reduce withdrawal symptoms and cravings without producing intoxicating effects.

STIMULANTS

- *Bupropion* (Zyban, Wellbutrin): reduces cravings for meth.

- *Modafinil* (Provigil, Alertec, Modavigil): used to treat sleeping disorders, but shown to reduce cocaine cravings and withdrawal symptoms.

OPIOIDS

- *Buprenorphine* (Subutex): reduces cravings and eases withdrawal symptoms, must be administered by a licensed and trained physician.

- *Methadone*: inhibits the effect of heroin and morphine, but can be administered only at a licensed clinic.

- *Naltrexone* (Ravia): (above).

- *Buprenorphine + naloxone* (Suboxone): used for maintenance therapy.

Chapter 6

Painless Detox

The process of detoxifying from alcohol or drug addiction is seared into the public conscience through popular culture. Even in the earliest days of cinema, movie producers grasped the drama associated with alcoholism and drug addiction. The 1902 French film *The Victims of Alcoholism* was the first feature in a string of Silent Era movies on both sides of the Atlantic to underscore the dangers of substance addiction and its withdrawal. In 1917, Charlie Chaplin jumped on the wagon with *The Cure* (1917), a film he directed and starred in about an upper-crust fop (a departure from his trademark tramp character), who causes mayhem when he arrives at a fancy hotel/spa resort, seeking help with his alcohol addiction, with a case of booze.

Chaplin had personal experience with the subject matter; his alcoholic father died at thirty-eight years old of cirrhosis of the liver. Although tackling serious social issues with humor—abject poverty, child abandonment, racism, prostitution—was a hallmark of Chaplin's films, in reality, detoxing from alcohol and drugs, until recently, was a horrifying process resulting in extreme physical pain, anxiety, depression, and even psychosis.

Today, the advent of new pharmaceuticals has made the process virtually pain free. However, because alcohol and opiate drugs (heroin, cocaine, prescription painkillers) affect different receptors in the brain, their detoxification must be administered with different techniques.

Research studies and my own extensive clinical experiences have shown a high success rate in treating alcoholics while they go cold turkey with benzodiazepines along with gabapentin, topiramate, and clonidine. For opiate detox, the preferred pharmaceutical is clonidine, supplemented with muscle relaxers, antinausea drugs, and other medications. However, don't try this at home! Detox from a severe addiction without proper *medical* supervision can result in brain damage and death.

Severe Intoxication and Detoxification

The American Society of Addiction Medicine lists three immediate goals for detoxification of alcohol and other substances: (1) "to provide a safe withdrawal from the drug(s) of dependence and enable the patient to become drug-free," (2) "to provide a withdrawal that is humane and thus protects the patient's dignity," and (3) "to prepare the patient for ongoing treatment of his or her dependence on alcohol or other drugs."

Detoxification for those in severe intoxication because of

alcohol, opiates (heroin and painkillers), stimulants (cocaine, meth), benzodiazepines (Xanax, Valium), and/or barbiturates can be fatal, and each patient must receive personalized medical care. Opiate withdrawal is very physically uncomfortable. Seizures, while common in the withdrawal process, are not usually fatal.

Extreme stimulant intoxication can precipitate symptoms similar to those of heart attacks and can cause strokes, seizures, arrhythmia, or life-threatening hyperthermia. The nonmedical use of methamphetamine has severe destructive potential for the brain, including microstrokes, neurotransmitter dysregulation, and death of brain cells. The long-term psychosis resulting from extreme and continued nonmedical use of methamphetamine is often misdiagnosed as schizophrenia. There are no life-threatening withdrawal considerations when someone stops using stimulants, although there is a crash period of exhaustion, lethargy, and depression.

Treating the Unique Addict or Alcoholic

As with all aspects of addiction treatment, detoxification must be individualized for each patient. No two people are the same, and each must receive a thorough medical evaluation before being given the appropriate medical care in a compressive program incorporating all the therapeutic and/or curative methodologies available.

In the previous chapter I mentioned that I usually avoid giving patients stimulants unless it turns out that they have undiagnosed attention deficit disorder (ADD). In the majority of those cases, once they are prescribed the most effective stimulant, their life is changed, and their drug misuse ends. For some diagnosed ADD patients who have a nonmedical stimulant dependence, even prescription stimulants trigger a relapse.

The point is this: Physicians need to keep an open mind and provide individualized treatment. The old belief that individual addicts are not different from each other is completely wrong. No two are exactly alike, and there is no one treatment that is appropriate for all patients. To overlook the individuality of the patient is a gross violation of both ethics and professional responsibility.

Detox vs. Treatment

Detox and treatment in the public's mind are synonymous, but in reality, that's not the case. Not every addict who seeks treatment needs to go through detoxification. It's only necessary for those patients whose dependence on a substance has reached such a critical stage that a sudden cessation—going cold turkey—could seriously endanger their health and possibly their lives.

This is the inherent problem in addiction rehab clinics that rely exclusively on nonmedical protocols and apply a one-size-fits-all abstinence model for treatment.

Detoxification is the removal of alcohol or other drugs from the body via metabolism and specifically through the liver and excretion through the kidneys. Medically assisted detoxification reduces the risk of discomfort and potential physical harm for patients in the throes of withdrawal. For those with severe substance dependency, detoxification is an often necessary step before moving on to immediate care and eventual long-term management of the disease of addiction.

Beside the fallacy that addiction treatment can be the same for everyone, another point of confusion needs to be cleared up: Detoxification is not the end of treatment but rather the precursor to it. I am reminded again of the death of actor Philip Seymour Hoffman. He reportedly checked himself into a detox center after a relapse in his drug addiction. He was released after ten days. In a few days he was back to shooting heroin and overdosed a few months later.

In my opinion, the ten-day detox, which has become a cultural ritual for the rich and famous, is more of a publicity stunt than bona fide medicine. When a celebrity gets in trouble and his career is in jeopardy, the knee-jerk response from his handlers is to exhort, "get thee to detox." That's like bandaging the wounds of a gunshot victim and then showing him the door.

The Three Steps to Detox

As outlined in the landmark addiction report known as the Columbia University CASA Report, published in 2014, there are three main components to effective detoxification. I use these in my own clinical practice.

1. EVALUATION

Examine the patient and determine if symptoms are acutely present, ideally using standardized instruments to measure the severity of withdrawal. Assess vital physical signs that manifest themselves in substance dependency. Evaluate for the presence of cooccurring medical conditions and mental health disorders. And, finally, determine by medical analysis, such as a urine test, if there are substances present in the patient's body or if substances were recently used.

2. STABILIZATION

The doctor and other trained personnel assist the patient through withdrawal to the state of physiological stability. Depending on the individual, pharmaceutical medications may be needed.

3. FACILITATION OF TREATMENT ENTRY

Guide patients with severe addiction to a bona fide addiction treatment center that uses evidence-based medicine and provides a continuation for the short-term care *and* long-term management of the patient's disease.

Alcohol Detoxification

Alcohol withdrawal is potentially the most dangerous of any substance addiction. For the successful and safe cessation of alcohol ingestion I recommend the use of certain medications to help prevent the harmful effects that may accompany it. Withdrawal from alcohol typically takes seven to ten days, but with medical management, stabilization can be achieved sooner.

During the first six to forty-eight hours, symptoms can include anxiety, nausea, agitation, and difficulty concentrating. In more severe cases, symptoms can include hallucinations and seizures. Alcohol withdrawal delirium, also known as delirium tremens (DTs), is the most severe and dangerous withdrawal symptom, and usually appears two to four days after the last drink. Some symptoms of alcohol withdrawal, including DTs and seizures, can be life-threatening, so it is medically imperative that patients severely addicted to alcohol should undergo detox only with the supervision of trained medical personnel with ready access to hospital care if necessary.

There are a number of assessment tools that can be used to determine the severity of alcohol addiction, including Clinical Institute Withdrawal Assessment—Alcohol Revised (CIWA-Ar), the Clinical Opiate Withdrawal Scale (COWS), and the Finnegan Neonatal Abstinence Score.

The duration of detoxification varies with the severity of addiction. Withdrawal symptoms, such as sleep disturbances, can last for weeks. The severity of symptoms can increase in patients who have experienced prior alcohol detoxifications, a process known as the kindling effect.

Here's the good news: As I mentioned before, benzodiazepines, a class of psychoactive tranquilizers, have calming, sedating effects and can prevent the onset of certain alcohol withdrawal symptoms and acutely relieve such symptoms, including alcohol-induced seizures and DTs. This class of drugs includes the following drugs (brand names in parentheses):

- Diazepam (Valium)
- Clonazepam (Klonopin)
- Lorazepam (Ativan)
- Chlordiazepoxide (Librium)

Because the combined effects of benzodiazepines and alcohol can be life threatening, patients must be advised not to drink while on benzodiazepine medications. Also, benzodiazepines have their own potential for addiction and so should be used only in the relatively short-term period of detoxification and closely monitored by a medical professional.

Although DTs occur only in about 5 percent of patients undergoing alcohol detoxification, the mortality rate is more than 18 percent for those who experience them. There's no excuse for anything but expert medical care for patients experiencing DTs.

Opioid Detoxification

Withdrawal symptoms from illicitly obtained or prescription opioids, including heroin, morphine, hydrocodone, and oxycodone, are not typically life threatening, but they can be extremely uncomfortable. Among the symptoms are abdominal pain, muscle aches, agitation, diarrhea, dilated pupils, insomnia, nausea, runny nose, sweating, and vomiting.

Withdrawal symptoms generally last from seven days to several weeks. Because medical complications can develop, patients must undergo regular physical examinations and psychological evaluations.

The goal of medical detoxification is a safe, comfortable and complete withdrawal from opioids. Sudden cessation of opioids, especially for a patient who has developed physical dependence on the drug, should be avoided. Rather, the patient should be weaned off the opioid gradually.

However, this procedure is not legally permissible with illicit opioids such as heroin.

Instead, the trained medical professional uses opioid replacement therapy, which substitutes FDA-approved medications that are then gradually tapered off. Nonopioid medications, such as clonidine, can decrease the agitation and discomfort associated with withdrawal. Other medications that can relieve the symptoms of acute withdrawal can also be used, such as nonsteroidal anti-inflammatory drugs (NSAIDs) to treat muscle pain, antiemetics for nausea, nonaddicting sleeping medications like trazodone for insomnia, and buprenorphine to stop the craving.

Medically prescribed opioids formulated specifically for addiction treatment work by occupying the opioid receptors in the brain, blocking or minimizing the effects of more addicting opioid drugs. A patient using buprenorphine is protected from inadvertent overdose and prevented from getting high.

Stimulant Detoxification

Detoxification from stimulants like cocaine and meth may result in withdrawal symptoms, but normally these symptoms are less severe than with alcohol and are rarely life threatening. Symptoms include lethargy, insomnia, agitation, anxiety, increased appetite, depressed moods, and drug cravings.

As with alcohol and substance detox, the preferred method is tapering the drug off gradually. But as with illicit opioids, stimulants like cocaine are illicit and cannot be used in detoxification. Tranquilizers can be used for agitation and anxiety, and nonaddictive sedatives are helpful with insomnia.

As noted in the previous chapter, there is promising evidence supporting a medication called bupropion for curbing cravings and reducing the severity of withdrawal symptoms associated with meth addiction. Bupropion was developed to treat depression, including seasonal affective disorder, and has been proven to aid in quitting smoking. The drug appears to work by blocking the receptors of two neurotransmitters active in substance addiction: dopamine and nor-epinephrine. Another advantage is that it curbs the increased weight gain associated with stimulants withdrawal.

Similarly, the stimulant medication modafinil (brand names Provigil, Alertec, and Modavigil), created to treat sleeping disorders, can reduce the cravings and withdrawal symptoms associated with cocaine. Studies are inconclusive as to modafinil's effectiveness, but depending on the individual patient, it can reduce the stimulating effects of cocaine and aid in overall detoxification.

Depressant Detoxification

Benzodiazepines are commonly known as tranquilizers and are some of the most commonly prescribed medications in the United States. Brands like Valium and Xanax are household names and are found in tens of millions of medicine cabinets across the country.

Xanax, designed for anxiety, is the most commonly prescribed pill in the United States, with nearly 48 million prescriptions written in 2012. When used as prescribed, benzodiazepines can help in legitimate medical conditions, such as anxiety, insomnia, seizure control, and muscle relaxation. Indeed, earlier in this chapter we learned how benzodiazepines can be effective in alcohol withdrawal.

It's when benzos are taken recreationally for their sedative effect that they cross the line into substance abuse.

Here's the shocker: They're as popular for their illicit use as they are for their legitimate use. Nearly 15 percent of Americans aged twenty-one to thirty-four have taken tranquilizers without a prescription or recreationally according to 2012 data from the Substance Abuse and Mental Health Services Administration.

There's even a sinister side to their abuse. Benzodiazepines are the so-called date rape drug, which can impair normal brain functions to the point that a person cannot resist, or even want to resist, sexual aggression.

Withdrawal from benzos is similar to that for alcohol, with seizures and delirium being the most serious side effects. Symptoms can last between one and two weeks. Because benzos are legal, a detox program can use the drug itself to slowly wean the patient from it. Alternately, a different benzo drug from the same class can be used for detoxification.

Detoxification Venues

Where detoxification takes place depends on the severity of the patient's addiction and overall health condition. Physicians' offices, mental health treatment facilities, urgent care centers, hospitals, ER departments, and even patients' homes can be appropriate once a proper assessment has been made of the nature of the detox required and, most important, if medical assistance is needed.

On the other hand, the worst detox scenario is having an addict sent to a so-called rehab clinic without medically trained personnel or one that outright rejects evidence-based medicine for addiction treatment; these facilities are often called "12-step recovery programs" or a variation on that theme. In other words, they are making a profit on the philosophical teachings of AA, which was always meant to be free, and offering no medical safeguards in the potentially dangerous detox process.

Patients most at risk are those with a history of severe withdrawals or multiple withdrawals. It's bordering on the criminal and is certainly unethical to place one of these patients in a nonmedical setting for detoxification.

As If They Were Never Treated

If there's one message to take away from this chapter, it's this: Medications offer help in suppressing withdrawal symptoms during detoxification; however, detoxification is not in itself a full treatment program. For addicts to believe their treatment program ends at evacuating the addictive substances from their body is nothing more than wishful thinking. Rather, it is only the beginning of the treatment process.

Patients who go through withdrawal—including medically assisted withdrawal—but who do not receive any further treatment, mimic drug abuse patterns similar to those who were never treated. It's as if they were never detoxed at all.

Licensed Medical Professionals

In this book I've stressed the need for addicts with a severe substance abuse, particularly with opioids and alcohol, to have their detoxification supervised by trained medical personnel, optimally a trained physician. Unfortunately, this is a small elite group whose ranks need to be greatly expanded.

As of 2015, the American Medical Association (AMA) estimated that of the 985,375 active physicians, there were only 582 addiction physician specialists: 227 addiction medicine physicians and 355 addiction psychiatrists—the two medical subspecialties specifically trained in addiction science and its treatment—totaling 0.06 percent of all active physicians.

Although there are no recent data identifying the actual number of practicing specialists in addiction medicine or addiction psychiatry, the American Board of Addiction Medicine has certified 2,584 addiction medicine specialists and estimates that the number of full-time practicing addiction medicine specialists may be about five times the number of the AMA estimate, or approximately 1,200. This estimate still falls far short of the estimated minimum of 6,000 full-time addiction medicine specialists currently needed to meet addiction treatment demands.

All opioid maintenance therapy facilities are required by federal law to obtain certification from the U.S. Department of Health and Human Services' Substance

Abuse and Mental Health Services Administration (SAMHSA) to demonstrate compliance with established standards for opioid maintenance therapy programs. It is a prerequisite of certification that a program be accredited by an organization approved by SAMHSA.

Becoming qualified to prescribe and distribute buprenorphine involves an approved eight-hour program in treating addiction, an agreement that the physician and medical practice will not treat more than 30 patients for addiction involving opioids with buprenorphine at any one time within the first year and up to 100 thereafter, and assurance that the trained physician will refer patients to necessary supplemental psychosocial services.

Physicians who meet the qualifications are issued a waiver by the SAMHSA and a special identification number by the Drug Enforcement Agency.

The key to finding evidence-based detoxification is to look for programs supervised by medical doctors or psychiatrists with board certification in addiction medicine by the American Board of Addiction Medicine.

Chapter 7

Maintenance and Relapse

ddiction is not a disease you can treat with a shot and be done with it. It's not the flu. It's a chronic disease, which, by definition, means there's no cure. Again, think heart diseases, asthma, and diabetes as reference points. Once the disease is stabilized, it must be treated over a lifetime.

As with any chronic disease, a degree of patient relapse is to be expected. The disease flares up, and you have to start the treatment again. Relapse is part of what having a chronic disease means—whether its hypertension or drug addiction. In fact, the relapse rate for addiction is typical of chronic diseases, slightly more than diabetes but less than hypertension and asthma.

A relapse is not an occasion to scold, punish, or otherwise stigmatize the person. It's not a moral failure but a symptom. Modern-day diagnostics indicate that most brains eventually return to relatively normal when the drug use stops. However, the neurological and psychological after-effects of drug use persist, and they make a relapse a significant possibility for months, years, even decades after initial treatment.

A single act can instantly reignite addiction pathways, causing the former addict to renew drug-seeking behavior. In effect, the addict's brain remembers that the substance—alcohol, cocaine, meth, Vicodin, bath salts, you name it—relieves stress, no matter how much time has passed.

The key to successful sobriety is regular, quarterly wellness checkups with a medical professional trained in addiction medicine, who can monitor brain chemistry, particularly neurotransmitter levels. Therapy and counseling can also assist in maintaining a lifestyle that avoids people and places that provide potential relapse triggers.

The Changing Face of the Addict

Knowing who suffers from the disease of addiction is essential for marshaling limited resources, both on a personal and societal level, and tailoring programs that best fit the most common profiles. A patient's demographic profile also can affect treatment. Women, for example, react differently from men to the same dosage of many drugs. Older patients absorb drugs differently from the population at large (age affects changes in body composition; the elderly typically have an increase in adipose tissue, decrease in lean body mass, decrease in total body water and lower metabolisms than the adult population at large).

Yet, the popular concept of who is an addict in America in the twenty-first century is woefully out of balance with reality.

The term *addict* still conjures up ideas of heroin junkies shooting up in a burned-out tenement in the Bronx. In reality, the drug addict today is likely to be a grandmother living in the suburbs who's hooked on prescription pills.

There's a whole new population of addicts unthinkable a generation ago, the so-called accidental addicts. They are fifty years old or older who may have started using a prescription drug to relieve legitimate pain, perhaps from one or more chronic conditions. Unfortunately, many of these patients inadvertently have formed a severe drug dependency. They now find themselves needing to ingest more and more of the painkiller simply to navigate their daily lives. In other words, they're addicted. From a pharmacological perspective, that's not surprising. Chemically speaking, there's a fine line between an illegal opioid like heroin and a legal opioid like hydrocodone.

In 2012, adults aged forty-five to sixty-four had the highest rate of hospital stays for opioid abuse; twenty years ago, that distinction belonged to those twenty-five to forty-four years old. More than 5.7 million people over the age of fifty will need substance abuse treatment by the year 2020, according to government researchers.

Heroin vs. Prescription Drugs

Without a doubt, there has been a dangerous resurgence in the use of heroin. Between 2012 and 2013, heroin overdose deaths in the United States soared by 39 percent from 5,925 to 8,257. Add deaths related to meth, cocaine, PCP, bath salts, Flakka, and every other illicit drug, and the best data shows they were responsible for approximately 16,000 deaths in 2014.

However, the much bigger problem is the abuse of prescription pills. Overdose deaths from controlled prescription drugs have increased significantly over the last decade and now surpass the number of overdoses caused by all illicit drugs combined, accounting for more than 38,000 deaths in 2010. Enough prescription painkillers were prescribed that year "to medicate every American adult around-the-clock for a month," according to the Centers for Disease Control and Prevention (CDC).

To frame the problem another way, healthcare professionals wrote 259 million prescriptions for painkillers in 2012. Which demographic group was impacted most by this tidal wave of opioid drugs? Seniors!

More than one-third of the enrollees in Medicare Part D, which covers the cost of pharmaceutical drugs for seniors, used a prescription opioid. In 2011, 11.5 million Medicare beneficiaries, who by definition are at least sixty-five years old, filled at least one prescription for an opioid analgesic (painkiller), collectively spending more than $2.7 billion.

The rates of patients dying from prescription opiate overdose deaths for those aged fifty-five to seventy-four increased about sixfold between 1999 and 2013, according to CDC statistics, even as all other age groups saw the rate of increase slow or stabilize.

If there is a silver lining in the prescription pill epidemic, it seems that beginning in 2010, it began to peak. Most experts attribute that to new restrictions on doctors from dispensing prescription pills. Unfortunately, and it appears not coincidentally, about the same time prescription pill use, or at least abuse, was beginning to decline, heroin use started to surge. Do you see the connection? With prescription pills increasingly hard to find and expensive on the black market, users began to turn to cheap heroin.

To add to the perfect storm, the new forms of heroin that have become available since about 2000 are so pure that they no longer have to be injected. The very stigma that had once defined the heroin junkie—shooting up (or intravenous injections)—was no longer necessary. Indeed, a study published in 2014 in the prestigious *JAMA Psychiatry* journal found that "80 percent of the people who had used heroin in 2010 had also used prescription pills," and that these users turned to heroin because it was "more readily accessible and much less expensive than prescription opioids."

Needless to say, the new users of heroin weren't kids but were older adults. Studies have shown that the face of the heroin user has changed over the last twenty years from young men in urban environments to older men and women located more in the suburbs.

The rate of death by accidental drug overdose for forty-five- to sixty-four-year-olds increased more than 10 times between 1990, when baby boomers were still outside the age group and 2010, when they were starting to fill the ranks of that age group. For the first time ever, deaths from accidental overdoses for late-middle-age adults exceeded those of the twenty- and thirty-somethings. In 2013, more late-middle-agers died from accidental overdoses than from car accidents or from the flu or pneumonia for that matter.

Dependence vs. Addiction

Emotional stress (psychological factors) can trigger the onset of a disease, including the disease of addiction, because stress may activate the genetic, biological factor. Stress may also trigger the relapse of a disease in remission.

People often confuse addiction with physical dependence in the context of clinical treatment. Drugs that we often associate with abuse, such as opiates or central nervous system stimulants, are, in the proper context, beneficial medications.

Addiction is also not synonymous with recreational or social use of mood-altering agents, including alcohol. Once we clear up this misunderstanding, everyone understands why addiction is a true clinical illness and why addiction is classified as a disease by every clinical organization in the world, including the AMA, the World Health Organization, and the American Psychiatric Association. Obviously, if addiction were not a clinical condition meeting the clear definition of disease, my area of specialization—addiction medicine—wouldn't exist.

Now, let us suppose that you use cocaine, or another stimulant, and have used it regularly for several years. Stimulants such as cocaine can contribute to, or precipitate, stroke, seizure, heat arrhythmia, heart attacks, and hyperthermia (a potentially fatal elevation of temperature). You go to the doctor for a checkup, and he tells you that because of the cumulative effect of your years of cocaine use, you must stop immediately or you will definitely have a heart attack or stroke. What do you do? Simple, you stop.

For most people, stopping heavy drinking or drugging, or other life-threatening behavior, is simply a decision they make in their own best interest. They might do so with the help of a psychologist, their primary care doctor, a family member or friend, a self-help group, or entirely on their own.

Most people who develop a substance dependency can simply end their habit. Because of all the consequences to their health and the safety of others and for the sake of their friends and families, their own financial well-being, their spiritual or philosophical beliefs, and their own sense of self and personal convictions, they choose to stop drinking or drugging excessively or altogether.

A Question of Choice

For the unlucky with the disease of addiction, it's not a question of choice. They can't simply stop taking their favorite drug (including alcohol). Likewise, they can't simply stop from relapsing.

Those scientifically proven facts about substance addiction still vex most Americans. They see addicts drinking and drugging, they know they themselves occasionally indulge in recreational drinking or drugging, and they know they can stop whenever they like. So, why can't addicts? If they just chose to stop, they wouldn't have their disease. It's so intuitive that it is hard to shake the idea that there's an alternative explanation.

Let's remove the stigma of addiction from the discussion for a moment. Many people know they have high cholesterol and high blood pressure, but make no attempt to control them. Finally, they have a heart attack or stroke. That is their choice. Many diabetics are not taking medication, cheat on their diet, and are walking around with sky-high blood sugar levels. Again, that is their choice. People choose to have unprotected sex, share needles, and possibly contract HIV/AIDS. Would you say that they chose to get HIV? No, but their choices facilitated the disease.

Can a person make a poor choice by drinking heavily knowing they have a strong family history of addiction? Yes, and that choice can lead to alcoholism, which is a form of addictive disease. The disease of addiction is, in many ways, similar to high blood pressure. People can't control their blood pressure by force of will or decision. People with the disease of addiction can't control their disease by force of thought. Patients with drug and alcohol addiction want to stop, but they need professional clinical help and true understanding from friends.

Addiction Defined by ASAM

Addiction is a primary, chronic disease of brain reward, motivation, memory, and related circuitry. Dysfunction in these circuits leads to characteristic biological, psychological, social, and spiritual manifestations. This is reflected in an individual pathologically pursuing reward and/or relief by substance use and other behaviors.

Let's recap: Addiction, according to the American Society of Addiction Medicine (ASAM), is characterized by the inability to consistently abstain, by impairment in behavioral control, by cravings, by diminished recognition of significant problems with one's behaviors and interpersonal relationships, and by a dysfunctional emotional response.

The ASAM Patient Placement Criteria focus on six dimensions to define severity: (1) potential for acute intoxication and/or withdrawal, (2) biomedical conditions and complications, (3) emotional/behavioral conditions or complications, (4) treatment acceptance/resistance, (5) relapse potential, and (6) recovery environment.

In the maintenance phase of treatment, the goal is to match the patient's needs to the appropriate service by assessing the severity of the addiction as well as verification of the medical diagnosis.

Managed Maintenance

Contrary to what many rehab clinics promote, there is no thirty-day fix for addiction (pardon the pun!). You can't permanently stop the progression of alcohol or drug addiction during a one-month stay any more than you could with diabetes or heart disease. Successfully treating addiction requires long-term medical intervention by trained professionals who can supervise and coordinate all treatment options.

There is no one-size-fits-all, long-term maintenance protocol for addiction treatment. Each patient's case is different, so maintenance and the recovery from inevitable relapses must be individualized.

Most addicts require additional pharmaceutical and psychological intervention after their conditions are stabilized. As discussed in the previous chapter, the measure of success for addiction treatment is not simply abstinence, which is the result of successful treatment. Rather, success is determined—as with all chronic diseases—by the quality of life. With medically supervised disease management, can the addict live a relatively normal and productive life?

I have had patients whose disease management and maintenance have lasted a few months after their initial condition has been stabilized. For other patients, I have been maintaining their health with a combination of medications and psychological counseling for years. The benchmark—the only measure of success—is their continued high quality of life.

For most patients, long-term managed care mimics in many ways the treatment provided during the acute care stage, which stabilized their condition. So, for example, a patient with an opioid addiction treated with the medication naltrexone in acute care would continue with that medication during the long-term maintenance of his treatment. Over time, the dosage of the medication would be reduced until the point when it would be no longer needed to diminish the patient's cravings for his addiction.

A new generation of extended-release naltrexone, sold under the brand name Vivitrol, is especially helpful in preventing relapse of opioid addicts. A study published in 2013 in the journal *Addiction* confirms what I was already seeing in my clinical experience: Vivitrol blocks the effects of the opioids (heroin was the focus in the study) on brain receptors and prevents relapse by reducing "euphoria, pain relief, sedation, physical dependence and cravings." That Vivitrol is injected once a month, rather than taken as a daily pill as with standard-release naltrexone, also circumvents the need for the patient to closely and constantly manage medications.

Ongoing psychosocial therapy would provide the patient with mechanisms for coping with stress and other situations that might trigger a flare-up of the disease. An overall health regimen of good nutrition and regular exercise would further reduce stressors that might cause a relapse.

Extreme Addiction Cases

Managed maintenance is a program with proven success in restoring health, life, and hope to those unique individuals who, because of either systemic or acquired medical conditions, have become completely dependent on opiate pain relievers. These special cases are patients with addiction histories, ten-to fifteen-year medical condition such as hepatitis C, HIV, heart problems, and/or psychiatric complications. These cases are not the norm, but not being a "normal" addict is no reason to be denied effective life-saving, health-restoring treatment.

Without managed maintenance, 80 percent of these extreme cases immediately fall right back into dangerous addiction. An addiction medicine specialist knows the proper and effective way to replace dangerous and illegal substances with FDA-approved Suboxone, a prescription medication also used in detox that keeps patients from experiencing life-threatening, debilitating withdrawal and allows them to remain physically stable.

Heroin Dependence

Previously, I noted how an advantage of Suboxone, a medication used in the treatment of heroin addiction, is that no tolerance developed, but there is a ceiling on the drug's effect. In other words, if you take more than your required amount, you won't get more high. Suboxone is available only by prescription and administered only by a physician.

Other advancements include new treatments for opioids and stimulants. For opioids, this includes long-acting injectable or implanted naltrexone, and antagonists; oral or implanted buprenorphine, a partial agonist; and innovative detoxification methods using buprenorphine.

Cocaine Dependence

New developments for cocaine dependence include vaccines that provide either active or passive immunization, agonists that could decrease craving without producing euphoria, blocking agents that do not block normal pleasures, and corticotrophin-releasing factor (CRF) antagonists that could decrease both craving and relapse. In the short term, modafinil, tiagabine, topiramate, and disulfiram, medications currently marketed for other conditions, show promise for cocaine addiction.

Psychiatric Realities

Failure to address psychiatric realities dooms a person to unnecessary consequences. One of my patients had been active in Alcoholics Anonymous for many years. He would stay sober with little or no difficulty for ten months and then relapse. This pattern continued for years. Finally he sought medical help. As it turns out, he had bipolar disorder with a ten-month cycle. Every ten months, he would enter a manic phase, during which he would relapse. All it took to rectify this long-standing problem was a daily dose of a readily available prescription medicine.

If this man had been psychiatrically diagnosed in the first place, years of disappointment and feelings of failure could have been avoided.

With addiction, there is a significant impairment in executive functioning, which manifests in problems with perception, learning, impulse control, compulsivity, and judgment. People with addiction often exhibit a lower readiness to change their dysfunctional behaviors, despite mounting concerns expressed by significant others in their lives. They also display an apparent lack of appreciation of the magnitude of cumulative problems and complications.

However, addiction is more than a behavioral disorder. Features of addiction include aspects of behaviors, cognitions, emotions, and interactions with others, including:

- Excessive use and/or engagement in addictive behaviors at higher frequencies and/or quantities than the person intended, often associated with a persistent desire for, and unsuccessful attempts at, behavioral control.
- Excessive time lost in substance use or recovering from the effects of substance use and/or engagement in addictive behaviors, with significant adverse impact on social and occupational functioning (for example, the development of interpersonal relationship problems or the neglect of responsibilities at home, school, or work).
- Continued use and/or engagement in addictive behaviors, despite the presence of persistent or recurrent physical or psychological problems that may have been caused or exacerbated by substance use and/or related addictive behaviors.
- A narrowing of the behavioral repertoire focusing on rewards that are part of the addiction and an apparent lack of ability and/or readiness to take consistent action toward change, despite recognition of problems.

Over time, repeated experiences with substance use or addictive behaviors are not associated with ever-increasing reward circuit activity and are not as subjectively rewarding. Once a person experiences withdrawal from drug use or comparable behaviors, there is an anxious, agitated, and unstable emotional experience related to suboptimal reward and the recruitment of brain and hormonal stress systems. This response is associated with withdrawal from virtually all pharmacological classes of addictive drugs.

While addicts develop tolerance to the high, they do not develop tolerance to the emotional low associated with the cycle of intoxication and withdrawal. Thus addicts repeatedly attempt to create a high. But what they mostly experience is a deeper and deeper low. While anyone may *want* to get high, those with addiction feel a *need* to use the addictive substance or engage in the addictive behavior to try to resolve their uncomfortable emotional state or their physiological symptoms of withdrawal. People with addiction compulsively use even though it may not make them feel good.

Close monitoring of the behaviors of the individual and contingency management, sometimes including behavioral consequences for relapse behaviors, can contribute to positive clinical outcomes. Engagement in activities that promote personal responsibility and accountability, connection with others, and personal growth also contribute to recovery.

The qualitative ways in which the brain and behavior respond to drug exposure and engagement in addictive behaviors are different at later stages of addiction from those in earlier stages, indicating progression, which may not be overtly apparent. As is the case with other chronic diseases, the condition must be monitored and managed over time to

- Decrease the frequency and intensity of relapses.
- Sustain periods of remission.
- Optimize the person's level of functioning during periods of remission.

In some cases of addiction, medication management can improve outcomes. In most cases of addiction, psychosocial rehabilitation and ongoing care with evidence-based pharmacological therapy provide the best results. Chronic disease management is important for decreasing episodes of relapse and their impact.

Support Services

Because many addicts have often destroyed their lives by the time they get effective treatment, it's important to treat the whole person rather than just the disease. They may find themselves unemployed, homeless, needing childcare, facing criminal justice problems, and embroiled in family problems.

In addition to medication and psychosocial therapy, a long-term maintenance program might include support services such as family counseling, mental health care, supplementary medical care, housing and legal assistance, and vocational services.

A Late-in-Life Addict

My patient Augustus, or "Gus" as he prefers, isn't anyone's idea of a drug addict. A sixty-six-year-old family man with a loving wife, three children, and one grandchild, Gus was connected to the sea for his entire career. He joined the navy right out of high school, spending his twenties bumming around the Hawaiian Islands as deck crew on fishing charter boats. There was lots of drinking and drugging in those days, he recalled. "Doc, if you ever been on a fishing charter boat, you know they're really just an excuse for spending the day having a big party. Yeah, it's nice to catch a fish or two, but if that doesn't happen, it's just more of an excuse to get high. Now imagine doing that seven days a week," he told me when we first met.

You might surmise that Gus was a primary candidate for becoming an addict. But a remarkable thing happened when he was thirty-two-years old. He met his eventual wife, a school-teacher, and he decided to stop his dependency on alcohol and cocaine. "OK, to be honest, my wife had a lot to do with it. She gave me an ultimatum. You can continue to pretend you're still a kid out of the navy and party every day, or you can settle down and live happily ever after with me," he said.

They soon started a family, and he went on to having a suc-cessful maritime career, first as the captain of his own sports fish-ing charter boat, then eventually earning his Merchant Marine credential and his tugboat license. He capped his career as the captain of one of the first-respond boats that rescued the crew from the BP oil disaster in the Gulf of Mexico.

Then, the real trouble began. He retired at age sixty-five with a good pension and, of course, the benefits of Medicare. One of the first things he did was to get some badly need orthopedic surgery. A long career involving heavy physical labor had ground away his cartilage, and so, in quick order, he got joint replacement surgery for both hips. His surgeon prescribed him Vicodin, an opioid anal-gesic, for the postoperative pain. A year later, after his prescription ran out, he began buying it on the black market. "I was hooked. I knew I was hooked but I couldn't stop. It was no longer so much about the pain but just being able to function as a human being. Without my Vikes, I would get very anxious during the day and couldn't sleep at night," he said.

When prescription pills became hard to find on the street, he switched to heroin. "I never thought me, a grandfather for God sakes, would ever become a heroin junkie. Even when I was a young buck, I steered away from the stuff. That was what hoods and losers took. But this new stuff was so powerful you could just snort it. I think it would have been different, harder to rationalize using it, if I had to inject myself with a needle," he said.

Gus was motivated to change. He was just beginning his retirement and, with two new hips, figured that he had at least two good decades ahead of him to enjoy traveling with his wife, visiting his kids, and even doing some sports fishing. To stop his cravings for opioid, I prescribed a regimen of Vivitrol, a kind of extended-release naltrexone, which has had years of proven results. Now that he once again was mobile, I also put him on a regular regimen of exercise (walking, alternating with biking) and a whole-food diet, all to reduce stress that could trigger a relapse.

Today, three years later, his addiction is under control. He occasionally drinks but only moderately. "Doc, the days when I would get blind drunk or fall-down high are over. I've too much to live for to let drinking or drugging get in the way," he says.

How to Find a Bona Fide Treatment Center

Where I live and work in Los Angeles, the airwaves are filled with TV commercials from addiction centers that you'd swear sound like they know what they're doing. Some of them look absolutely beautiful—with beachfront views of the Malibu coastline, hot tubs, and gourmet dining.

For the most part, however, it's all window dressing. The sad fact is that 90 percent of all addiction treatment centers, also known as rehab clinics, offer no evidence-based medicine. Among the 10 percent that do, often it's limited to detoxification.

Despite the advances made in medically assisted treatment, the days when rehab was a program driven by enforced abstinence and 12-step meetings (such as Alcoholics Anonymous and Narcotics Anonymous) are, unfortunately, still with us. Most rehab clinics are staffed with drug counselors who have little to no training and often whose only qualification is that they are in recovery from their own alcohol or drug addiction.

How is the consumer supposed to find a legitimate treatment facility? You have to do your homework. Most patients, or their families, do more research buying a car than deciding on a treatment center.

Look for a facility in which every aspect of treatment is built on a solid scientific foundation and clinically proven to be effective in overcoming addiction. It is most important that all aspects of addiction treatment be under the direction of an addiction medicine specialist. This physician or psychiatrist (not a psychologist) is qualified to coordinate, assess, and make ongoing diagnoses and medically assisted treatments. (The American Board of Addiction Medicine has a list of bona fide physicians at www.abam.net.)

The modern treatment approach identifies specific problems that require specific types of attention. This means that the patient can be placed in the least intensive, safest level of care and specifically treated with strategies selected from a wide range of effective treatments best suited to that patient's individual condition and situation. If a clinic offers only one kind of treatment, and doesn't take into account the individual needs of the patient, this should be a red flag.

An effective treatment must help clients address, identify, and describe the personal meaning of their addiction. Are they self-medicating, filling up an inner emptiness, numbing feelings related to a trauma, or all of the above? Unless clients understand what they are actually doing on a deep level, they will chronically relapse. A responsible comprehensive treatment program takes all aspects into consideration for the ongoing health and well-being of the client.

A word of caution: Even seemingly helpful sources of information can be misleading. For example, the Substance Abuse and Mental Health Services Administration (SAMHSA), an agency with the federal Department of Health and Human Services, offers an online database to locate "treatment facilities in the United States or U.S.

Territories for substance abuse/addiction and/or mental health problems." The list is vetted, but only in the most superficial way. The facilities listed must meet local licensing requirements for rehab clinics, which vary wildly between states and, for the most part, are negligible. Also, these facilities have no oversight except that they qualify in the minimum way to charge third-party insurers. That's it. There's not even an attempt to screen for whether the services are medically sound.

In the greater Los Angeles area, for example, the SAMHSA locator database lists 700 facilities (Yes, 700!). But scanning through this overwhelming list, I can count on two hands the facilities that actually offer medically sound, evidence-based treatment programs.

Of the estimated 25 million Americans who are substance abusers, only 2 million receive any kind of treatment and only about 1 in 10 of those receive any kind of evidence-based treatment. The math is both shocking and discouraging. However, there is new hope that things are about to change for the better. The Affordable Care Act (a.k.a. Obamacare) has mandated the first-ever primary care benefit for substance-use disorders, which means the disease of addiction will be treated more like diabetes.

Also, addiction research and policy pioneer Thomas McLellan, former deputy drug czar for the Obama administration, has spearheaded the development of a program that aims to bring a rigorous, *Consumer Reports*–style of evaluation to the nation's thousands of rehab clinics. If his plan goes to fruition, the information would be accessible via a website and is already available in the Philadelphia area. Each facility would be judged on 10 criteria points, culled from scientific literature, including whether the facility can prescribe medicine, attend to physical health and educational hurdles, and prepare patients for a long-term recovery, including monitoring and support.

A Progressive Model for Treatment

Doctors become addicts, just like every other segment of the population. But physicians who become addicted present a particularly high risk to the public. One mistake in prescribing a medication, for instance, could kill a patient.

What happens to doctors who are addicted offers a template of treatment for the public at large. The Physician Health Program (PHP), used in all fifty states and the District of Columbia by medical societies and licensing boards, is more intensive and lasts longer than the treatment programs available on average by the general public. While thirty days is the average treatment for insurance-funded public programs, PHP offers a structured therapy lasting between three and six months, followed by five years of maintenance or managed care. The program, which is funded by grants and contributions for physicians, hospitals, and others interested in physical health issues, includes pharmaceutical and psychosocial therapy, nutrition and exercise counseling, and other support services (depending on the needs of the individual).

PHP's long-term monitoring has proven to reduce relapse. When relapses do occur, the response is therapeutic, not punitive. Studies have shown that physicians in the program who relapse tend to improve quickly after a treatment adjustment.

After five years more than 80 percent of the participating physicians return to work and remain substance free.

Chapter 8

Dual Diagnosis

In previous chapters we discussed the biological nature of addiction, the social and political currents that have shaped the disease in the public eye, and the changing demographics of those who suffer from it. But would you know an addict if you met one?

Let's take a typical social gathering of a hundred adults, say, at a wedding or a holiday office party. About nine of those there will regularly buy drugs illegally—opioids (heroin or prescription painkillers like Vicodin and OxyContin), stimulants (cocaine, meth, or bath salts), sedatives (Sizzurp, barbiturates), hallucinogens (ecstasy, LSD), tranquilizers (Valium, Xanax), or marijuana (legal in some states).

About ten will either be at high risk of becoming or already be an alcoholic, consuming an average of seventy-four drinks per week or the equivalent of eighteen bottles of wine—by themselves—per week. These heavy drinkers make up only 10 percent of the U.S. adult population, but are responsible for 60 percent of all alcohol sales (spirits, wine, and beer).

About half those at high risk for an alcohol or drug dependency actually suffer from an addiction, probably beginning early in their lives (more on that in the next chapter), although increasingly, beginning in late middle age (as we discussed in the last chapter). And a little over half of that subset will have a substance addiction *and* a diagnosable mental disorder (likely depression, but also possibly bipolar disease, schizophrenia, attention deficit hyperactivity disorder, autism, or psychosis).

So, if one in ten people have a substance addiction—the equivalent of the entire population of Texas—and a little more than half also have a mental disorder, could you pick those six people out among a hundred people in a room? Likely not. And that's a problem because as bad as treatment is in the United States for substance addiction in general, it's even worse for those addicted and mentally ill, a condition known as *dual diagnosis*.

Dual Diagnosis

I regularly see individuals with highly complex problems involving more than one diagnosis. They may have heart and liver problems, brain dysfunction, ulcers, plus psychological disorders, all in addition to an addiction to alcohol or drugs.

Most worrisome, however, is the correlation between mental illness and drug use that has been clearly established with about half of those with an alcohol or drug abuse problem showing signs of psychiatric disorder.

Dual diagnosis, also known as co-occurring disorder, is when a person is suffering from both the consequences of substance misuse and a simultaneous mood disorder, such as depression, bipolar disorder, panic disorder, or a more severe mental condition, such as schizophrenia.

There is a difference between induced psychosis from drugs or alcohol and psychosis as a result of mental illness. Induced psychosis is not uncommon, even with perfectly legal medications that affect brain chemistry. In that situation, the psychosis goes away as the drug's effects diminish over time. When the psychosis is the result of a mental illness, it does not diminish over time. It needs specific medical treatment.

When a patient has both drug-induced psychosis and mental illness, there are unique challenges to effective treatment. Even identifying both conditions presents problems. Drugs and alcohol can worsen the severity of mental disorders and present symptoms that look like those of mental disorders or, conversely, cover them up. Both severe intoxication and detoxification can give the appearance of mental illness, and vice versa.

It is so difficult to tell the difference that only 2 percent of mentally ill patients with substance abuse problems were detected in a university hospital emergency room. A state hospital did slightly better, detecting 15 percent.

Roughly 50 percent of individuals with severe mental disorders are affected by substance abuse, and 37 percent of alcohol abusers and 53 percent of drug abusers also have at least one serious mental illness. Of all people diagnosed as mentally ill, 29 percent also have problems with either alcohol or drugs. In those people diagnosed with bipolar disease, substance use problems are seven times more likely than for the nonbipolar population.

One recent study revealed that 33.7 percent of schizophrenics also meet the criteria for a diagnosis of alcohol use disorder, and 47 percent of individuals with schizophrenia are more than four times as likely as the general population to have a substance abuse disorder.

The Need for Specialized Care

A person with dual diagnosis needs specialized professional care, and most mental health services are not prepared for patients who also have severe drug and alcohol problems. As a result, the individual may be bounced back and forth between services for mental illness and those for substance abuse, or they may be refused treatment altogether. Many treatment centers will not take a person with dual diagnosis because they don't have qualified medical personnel on staff to deal with mental health issues.

A "traditional" or religious-centric nonmedical rehab is definitely not a good place for someone with a mental illness because these patients are very emotionally fragile and sensitive. Being placed in a confrontational, accusatory, and coercive environment can be the worst thing for them and for those around them.

Many patients who need medication for mental disorders have self-medicated with street drugs. They go to 12-step recovery support groups, where they are told they are not "clean and sober" if they are taking medically prescribed medication. This is not only absurd and cruel but a direct contradiction of the original

12-step philosophy, which allowed for psychiatric or psychological treatment whenever appropriate. There is even a brochure published by AA General Services, titled "A.A. Member—Medications and Other Drugs" that says members can take medications under a qualified physician's monitoring and that "no A.A. member should 'play doctor'" and offer unqualified medical advice to other members.

Unfortunately, there are few consequences for local AA groups that ignore that directive and impose a complete ban on medications, even pharmaceutical drugs prescribed by a physician for a mental disorder. This is all the more ironic since Bill W. (as he was known until after his death) conceived of AA after being treated at one of the first specialized addiction treatment hospitals in the country with a natural pain reliever that had known hallucinogenic effects, belladonna. In addition, he was exploring the use of a synthetic hallucinogen, LSD, as a possible treatment for alcohol addiction shortly before his death.

The dual-diagnosis patient is often discriminated against by nonmedical treatment professionals and emotionally abused by other recovering addicts and alcoholics who insist that all drugs are bad—often said while consuming massive amounts of caffeinated coffee and smoking cigarettes (which contain nicotine, a highly addictive stimulant drug). These unfortunate individuals find themselves as outcasts from both the drug and alcohol recovery community and from the mental health recovery community, and they are almost twice as likely to stop participating in outpatient mental health treatment than those who don't have issues with drugs and/or alcohol.

Integrating Treatment

Until recently, many mental health professionals believed that a patient with a dual disorder should be treated sequentially and that the substance addiction had to be cured before the mental disorder could be treated. There was a subtext to this approach that the addiction could be responsible for the mental disorder. To a degree, that was correct as it applied to drug- or alcohol-induced psychosis.

Today, we know that a nondrug or nonalcohol psychosis in a dual disorder is rare and that clinical depression is the most prevalent mental disorder. What, then, is the best approach to treating a dual diagnosis?

It is my opinion that the answer lies in integrating mental health and addiction treatment in a single, comprehensive program designed to meet the individual needs of the specific patient.

This approach is of proven value and is endorsed by Kathleen Sciacca, the founding executive director of Sciacca Comprehensive Service Development for Mental Illness, Drug Addiction, and Alcoholism in New York City. "There is a need for education that demonstrates that addictive disorders are illnesses," says Sciacca. "Understanding mental illness as a disease that is not caused by families was necessary to successful advocacy for the mentally ill. The same advocacy must happen for those who are dually diagnosed, through a clear understanding of the addictive disorders."

Distinguishing between Disorders

Even to the trained eye, the difference between dual pathology—addiction and mental disorder—and a mental disorder that has been substance induced can be elusive. Yet knowing the difference can have important implications for treatment. Because symptoms are similar, it's tempting to question whether all mental disorders suffered by addicts are induced by substance abuse. Yet, causative studies don't support the notion.

For example, public health surveys do not reflect a spike in the prevalence of dual disorder diagnoses when various drugs fall in and out fashion. That is, the recent rise in heroin addiction is not reflected in an increased incidence of pathological disorders among users. Simply put, exposure to addictive drugs does not increase mental illness, even though both can affect the brain similarly.

Identifying which is which remains a vexing problem for clinicians. There are diagnostic tools—tests to evaluate and assess the patient's mental health—that have been developed to help distinguish dual disorders from substance-induced disorders. These include Global Appraisal of Individual Needs—Short Screener (GAIN-SS) and Psychiatric Research Interview for Substance and Mental Disorders (PRISM) for the *Diagnostic and Statistical Manual for Mental Disorders*. However, by far the best diagnostic instrument is the *clinician's experience in treating addiction*, which speaks to the need for more doctors and health-care professionals trained in addiction medicine.

Substance-induced psychiatric symptoms can occur both in

the intoxicated state and during the withdrawal state. For instance, severe anxiety and depression are common symptoms among alcoholics. Even binge drinking can increase anxiety and depression levels in some individuals. And, more often than not, psychiatric disorders induced by prolonged alcohol or drug abuse will eventually disappear with proper treatment and a sustained period of abstinence.

It's worth noting that abuse of hallucinogens can trigger flashbacks, delusional and other psychotic phenomena that occur months or even years after stopping the use of the drug. The condition is most associated with an acid flashback, meaning LSD induced, but there have been anecdotal reports of former ecstasy users experiencing flashbacks as well.

When Drugs Meet Mental Illness

I met my patient Samantha forty-eight hours after she had passed out from overdosing on ecstasy at an all-night rave. After an initial exam, I observed that her condition was more than substance abuse and that she likely suffered from a mental disorder.

Samantha, twenty-four years old, was a production assistant in the wardrobe department for a prime-time TV show. Pretty and fashionable, she looked the part of young professional in Hollywood. She described her work as an "investment in her future," exciting at times, but mostly stressful.

"When we're in production, I have to be on call virtually any hour. There's no down time, and my days can last eighteen hours," she said.

She used electronic dance parties as her pressure valve. "They really are a great way to escape for a while. And Molly [ecstasy] just enhances the whole experience," she said.

Lately, however, she became aware that she might be using ecstasy too much. Over the preceding eight weeks there had been times when she attended raves and used the drug that she forgot what she had been doing for several hours. Her blackout incident two days before our first visit had scared her. "If I had not been with friends—really good friends—I don't know what would have happened. Fortunately, they were there and got me to an ER," she said.

While Samantha was abusing a drug, and an illegal one at that, she was not an addict. She limited her use of the drug to weekends. While there was no way of knowing for sure, one reason she passed out the last time she used ecstasy was likely because it had been mixed with another drug, perhaps a sedative. She admitted that she bought the ecstasy tablets the evening in question from a new dealer because she couldn't find her regular pill man.

In her case, she didn't have so much a drug dependency as a behavioral problem. Psychology counseling and lifestyle medication were the best therapies for her (besides, medication was not an option because there are no known pharmacological treatments for ecstasy addiction).

However, beyond her drugging, Samantha exhibited several signs that indicated she had clinical depression. Physically, she had a flat, emotionless tone to her voice and had a difficult time holding eye contact. She also reported having recurring insomnia. While she worked long hours during the week, she said that she was tired "all the time," even on weekends. Finally, she disclosed that her family had a history of bipolar disease.

I introduced her to cognitive behavioral therapy, a short-term counseling program that helps patients see how self-destructive behaviors can play a role in depression and comes up with strategies for avoiding those problems. Her treatment also included a regimen of meditation to deal with anxiety, a healthier diet, and techniques for avoiding insomnia.

Finally, I prescribed a medication known as a selective serotonin reuptake inhibitor (SSRI). The SSRIs include citalopram (Celexa), escitalopram (Lexapro), paroxetine (Paxil), fluoxetine (Prozac), and sertraline (Zoloft). Side effects are generally mild and, if taken under the close monitoring of a trained health professional, are both safe and effective.

Over the course of six months, Samantha steadily improved. I saw her every week for the first month and then once every two weeks for next three months. Then I saw her just monthly. That time when she passed out was the last time she used ecstasy, though she confessed to continuing to smoke pot on occasion. She no longer goes to raves but still enjoys seeing live music with her friends. And she quit her job and is now pursuing a master's degree in economic anthropology. "I finally figured out what I was passionate about, and it wasn't either fashion or Hollywood," she said.

Individualized Treatment

To overlook the individuality of a patient with dual disorder is likely not only to result in ineffective treatment but also is a gross violation of medical ethics and professional conduct. Because of both the complexity of the disease and the individuality required for its treatment, there is no simple one answer fits all treatment —in spite of what many rehab clinics would have you believe.

Despite the general consensus among medical professionals that those with dual diagnoses of addiction and mental illness must be treated for both conditions if they are to stay sober, very few rehab clinics, and even very few doctors, are trained to treat the afflicted.

Theories of Dual Diagnosis

The idea that all addicts are crazy and take drugs and alcohol in order to self-medicate is a popular notion, but one with only a kernel of truth. In fact, only about 50 percent of all addicts have a mental disorder.

Not all addicts who have a dual disorder take drugs to deaden their mental anguish. Addiction is mainly a condition of the brain in which the rewards circuitry is damaged—a physical condition that can be observed with diagnostic imaging, such as MRI.

The exact relationship between substance abuse and mental disorders is unknown. Until a unifying proven theory emerges, backed by research, there are a number of competing and complementary explanations for dual disorders.

Causality: This theory suggests that casual substance abuse may lead to mental illness. Cannabis is the focus of this research that hypothesizes even limited use of marijuana can significantly increase the risk of psychotic disorders like schizophrenia. However, proponents of the theory have failed to explain why the rates of schizophrenia and other psychoses have not increased despite a sharp upward trend in marijuana use over the last four decades (in 1969, 4 percent of the general population had tried marijuana; in 2013, 38 percent had).

Attention deficit hyperactivity disorder: One in four people who have a substance use disorder also have ADHD. Research has shown that ADHD is associated with an increased craving for drugs and that substance abuse results in more mental disorders than the population at large.

Autism spectrum disorder: Interestingly, while ADHD and autism have a strong correlation and share many of the same symptoms, they have the opposite effect in regard to substance abuse. While ADHD seems to increase the risk of addiction, autism decreases it. Some theorize that autism's inherent personality traits of inhibition and introversion act as a barrier against drug abuse. On the other hand, studies have shown that alcohol can worsen impaired social skills associated with autism, such as the ability to perceive emotions and understand humor.

Alleviation of dysphoria: Dysphoria is the opposite of euphoria (dysphoric feelings include anxiety, depression, boredom, and loneliness). This theory suggests that individuals with mental illness have a pronounced feeling of dysphoria, which prompts them to drink and drug to relieve their psychic pain. Scientific literature supports the idea that these feelings are a prime factor in substance abuse.

Multiple risk factors: This theory offers that there isn't just one primary cause of dual disorder but many, including such factors as poverty, peer pressure, dysfunctional childhood, sexual abuse, social isolation, and lack of structured daily activity (like employment).

Supersensitivity: In this theory, stress during childhood triggers inherent vulnerabilities (genetic and environmental) in the individual, rendering him supersensitive to the negative effects of alcohol and drugs. Later, exposure to even comparatively small amounts of alcohol or drugs can result in disproportionate negative effects, including violent, aggressive, and even criminal behavior.

PTSD, Vets, and Addiction

Post-traumatic stress disorder (PTSD) was not recognized as a mental illness until 1980. During World War I more than 300 "hysterical" soldiers—likely suffering from PTSD—were simply shot. During World War II they were branded cowards and during the Vietnam War, as schizophrenics.

Today, it's the most common psychiatric disorder among war veterans, including those from Vietnam, Iraq, and Afghanistan. With hundreds of thousands of soldiers returning from active duty in the last decade, there is a whole new wave of PTSD patients who also are addicts.

About 9 million vets are currently under Veterans Administration care, with 27 percent diagnosed with PTSD. Studies have shown there is a strong relationship in veterans between PTSD and a substance addiction, and about one-third of vets seeking treatment for addiction are also diagnosed with PTSD. In short, there are likely hundreds of thousands of vets suffering from the dual disorder of substance addiction and PTSD.

Unfortunately, the medications that work for one condition don't seem to work for the other.

The FDA-approved medications for PTSD, sertraline and paroxetine, have shown little benefit for treatment of substance use disorders. Similarly, the FDA-approved pharmacotherapies for alcohol dependence, naltrexone and disulfiram, have been shown to reduce alcohol dependence in veterans with PTSD but have not shown any particular benefit for PTSD.

The treatment of the co-occurrence of PTSD and substance addiction among veterans, as is the case with dual disorders with the populace at large, requires an individualized approach to treatment.

Chapter 9

Teens and Young Adults

n 1982, when then First Lady Nancy Reagan was asked by a schoolgirl what to do if she was offered drugs, she responded saying, "Just say no!"

Thus began a forty-year public relations campaign that, incredibly, in spite of its abject failure and $50 billion price tag, continues today. There's no evidence that the campaign has had any measurable effect on alcohol or drug addiction, and if anything, addiction among young people has gotten worse. Though it's no longer actively promoted, the Just Say No campaign, an offshoot of the larger war on drugs initiative, still influences politicians, educators, police authorities, and even the judiciary.

That an entire multibillion-dollar program to stymie youth addiction evolved not from research but from a knee-jerk phrase speaks volumes about the misplaced priorities and wasted resources of a nation. If anyone truly believes that tossing a throwaway phrase at kids is sound strategy for dealing with the drug culture all around them, then they must really think kids are stupid. And they're not.

The Just Say No campaign, the war on drugs, and virtually every other effort to stop teen addiction since Congress approved the Harrison Narcotics Act in 1914, including the now hilarious 1936 documentary film *Reefer Madness*, have failed because they don't pass the smell test: Their scare tactics and propaganda that any and all drinking and drugging lead to a straight and narrow path to addiction is false, and kids know it.

The Just Say No phrase, however, is not only useless but pernicious because it reinforces the false notion, promulgated by a well-intentioned AA community and exploited by the unscrupulous rehab industry, that addiction is simply something you can say no to. If you try hard enough, you can just stop. Addiction is like all other chronic diseases, including diabetes, heart disease, or arthritis. Just say no and you can just stop suffering from these diseases. (Oh, that's not right, is it?)

Addiction by the Numbers

Nine out of ten Americans who meet the medical criteria for addiction started smoking, drinking, or using other drugs before age eighteen, according to the national study "Adolescent Substance Use: America's #1 Public Health Problem," Columbia University's CASA study on addiction.

The CASA report finds that one in four Americans who began using any addictive substance before age eighteen are addicted, compared to one in twenty-five Americans who started using at age twenty-one or older.

Other relevant stats from the study:

- 75 percent (10 million) of all high school students have used addictive substances, such as alcohol, marijuana, and cocaine; one in five of them meets the medical criteria for addiction.

- 46 percent (6.1 million) of all high school students currently use addictive substances; one in three of them meets the medical criteria for addiction.

- 72.5 percent have drunk alcohol.

- 36.8 percent have used marijuana.

- 14.8 percent have misused controlled prescription drugs.

- 65.1 percent have used more than one substance.

The study found that, to a large degree, American culture drives teen substance use: "A wide range of social influences subtly condone or more overtly encourage use, including acceptance of substance use by parents, schools and communities; pervasive advertising of these products; and media portrayals of substance use as benign or glamorous, fun and relaxing."

These cultural messages and the widespread availability of alcohol, marijuana, and illicit and controlled prescription drugs normalize substance use, undermining the health and futures of our teens:

- 46 percent of children under age eighteen (34.4 million) live in a household where someone eighteen or older is smoking, drinking excessively, misusing prescription drugs, or using illegal drugs.

- 42.6 percent of parents list refraining from smoking cigarettes, drinking alcohol, using marijuana, misusing prescription drugs, or using other illicit drugs as one of their top three concerns for their teens.

- 21 percent say that marijuana is a harmless drug.

In addition to the heightened risk of addiction, the consequences of teen substance use include accidents and injuries; unintended pregnancies; medical conditions such as asthma, depression, anxiety, psychosis, and impaired brain function; reduced academic performance and educational achievement; criminal involvement; and even death.

If you don't care about the personal well-being of teenagers, then consider the costs to society:

- $14 billion in substance-related juvenile justice costs with teen substance use the origin of the largest preventable and most costly public health problem in America today.

- $68 billion in immediate costs per year of teen use, which includes an estimate associated with underage drinking and drugging.

- $468 billion per year in total costs to federal, state, and local governments of substance use that has its roots in adolescence.

- $1,500 per year is the cost for every person in America for teen substance abuse.

"The problem is not that we don't know what to do, it's that we are failing to act," noted Susan Foster, CASA's vice president and director of policy research and analysis. "It is time to recognize teen substance use as a preventable public health problem and addiction as a treatable medical disease, and to respond to it as fiercely as we would to any other public health epidemic threatening the safety of our children."

Why Treating Teenagers and Young Adults Is Different

It's no big secret that teenagers drink alcohol and do drugs. What's not understood by the public and even most medical professionals is why. Young people begin their quests for identity, for their sense of self, in their teen years. To be clear, teenagers base their self-identity entirely on how they see themselves, not on how their parents see them. Studies have shown that one primary way teens demonstrate their struggles with identity is indulging in forbidden behavior, including drinking and drugging, behaviors associated with adulthood.

Compounding the problem of teens' natural predilections to experiment with drugs and alcohol is that physiologically they are more sensitive to brain damage from addiction because their brains are still developing. Unfortunately, most efforts at teen addiction are rooted in the early twentieth-century doom-and-gloom philosophy, which most teens correctly perceive as irrelevant to their lives.

It's important to underscore, however, that not every teen who experiments with alcohol or drugs will become an addict; in fact, most will not. Maia Szalavitz, one of the nation's leading neuroscience and addiction journalists, pointed out in a recent column for Substance.com that the average cocaine addiction lasts four years, the average marijuana addiction lasts six years, and the average alcohol addiction is resolved within fifteen years. Heroin addictions tend to last as long as alcoholism, but prescription opioid problems, on average, last five years. A self-described addict who shot cocaine and heroin in her youth, she stopped when she was twenty-three years old, theorizing that, in effect, her brain finally grew up: "Although I got treatment, I quit at around the age when . . . the prefrontal cortex—the part of the brain responsible for good judgment and self-restraint—finally reaches maturity."

Truly successful teen addiction education and treatment are based on nonjudgmental harm-reduction programs, grounded in reality (not some war on drugs spin). Bottom line: The treatment for a binge-drinking teen must be entirely different from that of a middle-aged alcoholic with decades of continual consumption.

First, Do No Harm

If we are truly to reduce harm, we must give practical, short-term harm-reduction messages with which youth can identify and personalize. We have a much better chance of preventing a drunk-driving tragedy the night of the prom than we do preventing liver failure in forty years.

Writer, comic, and self-confessed screw-up Amy Dresner—known for her no-holds-barred skits that frequently incorporate references to her own personal addiction—recalls how she used to shoot meth directly into her bloodstream with a needle. As she did it more and more, she began having violent seizures. She rightly perceived the danger of possible traumatic brain injury during a meth-induced seizure. "I realized that shooting meth was an extreme contact sport requiring safety equipment," jokes Dresner. "I started wearing a football helmet when shooting up."

Silly as it sounds, Dresner was taking a positive step by considering and using the concept of harm reduction. She protected herself from a possible traumatic brain injury. The natural progression of harm-reduction thinking is to reduce harm as much as possible at all times and under all conditions. This leads to the realization of the need to stop the dangerous behavior. Dresner no longer shoots meth, and the football helmet is no longer required.

Preventing a drunk driving casualty can be accomplished by alerting teens to the real immediate danger of such behavior and by providing alternative transportation to and from parties and events. The obstacle to this life-saving strategy is that it requires dealing with reality, and harm-reduction strategies run into difficulty because they are predicated on dealing with the fact that many teens are already drinking.

As international researchers have noted, this is a major problem in the United States, where the uniform minimum legal drinking age is twenty-one, but the average age when people start drinking is thirteen or fourteen. This means that that alcohol education programs used in American schools start out with a major handicap: The erroneous assumption that a significant segment of the target audience is not already drinking or experimenting with drugs.

Peter E. Nathan, in his study "Alcohol Dependency Prevention and Early Intervention," cited research indicating that "students who are most responsive to school-based programs probably are those for whom such programs are least necessary. Programs may not be reaching those children who are at greatest risk to develop alcohol and drug problems."

In the high-risk category were teens with a family history of abuse, those with a history of antisocial behavior, and those from ethnic and racial minority groups who were "physically or psychologically beyond the reach of traditional, school-based prevention programs."

Successful programs use honest and effective educational strategies that treat drug use as just another part of a broad health curriculum that includes topics such as medical care, nutrition, exercise, hygiene, ecology, safety, and other activities that affect the students' quality of life.

In the prevention of addiction and alcoholism, addressing only drugs and alcohol overlooks other factors contributing to the onset of drug- and alcohol-related illness and addiction. An effective school program should send an honest, positive message that includes models beyond abstinence, embracing moderation, harm reduction, and personal responsibility. If possible, school-based prevention programs should be integrated into the school's academic program, because school failure is strongly associated with drug abuse. Integrated programs strengthen students' bonding to the school and reduce their likelihood of dropping out.

Any program used to prevent or reduce underage drinking and drug use must be continually evaluated. An evaluation needs to answer the following questions:

- What was accomplished in the program?
- How was the program carried out?
- How much of the program was received by participants?
- Is there a connection between the amount of program received and outcomes?
- Was the program run as intended?
- Did the program achieve what was expected in the short term?
- Did the program produce the desired long-term effects?

Repeated research and evaluation of successful methods shows that the most proven and practical approach for dealing with teen drinking and drug use is strategic harm reduction. In other words, make the world a safer place—safe *for* the drunk teen and safe *from* the drunk teen. Just as seat belts and airbags are harm-reduction strategies for road safety, the idea is to put a separation between the individual and harm, and society and harm.

Harm-reduction projects have aimed to minimize potential casualties and other damages associated with drinking in bars and nightclubs. Bars in the United States are now forbidden to serve alcohol to someone who is obviously intoxicated. They are also legally restrained from verbally encouraging people to get drunk. If a drunk driver kills someone and that driver was served alcohol when he was already drunk, the bartender may be criminally liable. While it can be argued that the person refused service will go elsewhere, it is hoped that his or her degree of intoxication will not increase.

Taking keys away from drunks and calling them a taxi to get them home is a major harm-reduction policy that is saving lives, as is the concept of the designated driver. "Friends don't let friends drive drunk" is a major harm-reduction campaign in the United States, and it is having a beneficial effect.

Reducing Harm

Harm reduction is a health-centered approach that seeks to reduce the health and social harms associated with alcohol and drug use, without necessarily requiring users to abstain.

Harm reduction is a nonjudgmental response that meets users where they are in regard to their substance use rather than imposing a moralistic judgment on their behaviors. This approach includes a broad range of responses, from those that promote safer substance use to those that promote abstinence.

The following features of harm reduction are clear indicators of why programs and campaigns based on this premise work:

- *Pragmatism:* Harm reduction accepts that some use of psychoactive substances is inevitable and that some level of substance use is expected in a society.
- *Humane values:* The substance user's decision to use alcohol and other drugs is accepted as his or her choice; no moralistic judgment is made, either to condemn or to

support use of substances, regardless of level of use or mode of intake. The dignity and rights of the person who uses alcohol and other drugs are respected.

- *Focus on harms:* The extent of a person's substance use is of secondary importance to the harms resulting from that use.
- *Hierarchy of goals:* Most harm-reduction programs have a hierarchy of goals; the symptoms that are the most potentially harmful to the patient are addressed first.

The Harm of Social Consequences

Interaction with a punitive law-enforcement system is also harmful. Research has shown that the risks associated with drugs other than alcohol are far less than those associated with alcohol, especially for those associated with aggression and violence. The punishment handed out for illicit drug use is more harmful than the drug use itself.

Due to the relatively low harm potential of cannabis, one important aspect of harm reduction would be to limit testing for cannabis use in those jurisdictions where testing positive for cannabis would result in harmful punitive actions because of existing laws.

For example, if a foreign exchange student in America under a federal program smokes pot at a party, and his host family finds out, they are obligated to report it. Once reported, the student is never allowed to pursue a college education or career in the United States nor can he or she ever enter America again. The harm was not done by smoking marijuana. The harm was done by the punishment.

None of these long-term concerns, be they consequences of health or punishment, has any meaning to a teenager who can't imagine life twelve months down the road, let alone the impact of current behavior on advanced educational opportunities, marriage, family, and employment in some distant future.

A successful technique for reducing the risk of teen drinkers becoming alcoholics is friendly advice offered to the heavily drinking teenager by someone he or she trusts. It is important that advice to moderate consumption not be confrontational or judgmental in any way. No criticism, no drama, no threats or stress. A very brief, simple moment of advice to reduce consumption and/or moderate behavior has proven far more motivating than lectures, scolding, or threats.

Removal of secrecy has also proven a powerful method. When teens are told by their own parents or guardians that if they really want to drink or drug, they are more than welcome to do it right there at home, the mystique of substance use being a secretive or rebellious act evaporates faster than alcohol.

Treating Teenagers and Young Adults

Teenage experimentation with alcohol and drugs is normative, no matter how much we pretend otherwise. In other words, it may not be healthy behavior, or behavior parents approve of, but it is normal behavior.

There are teens who excessively use drugs and alcohol, but actual teenage alcoholism is a rarity. There are thirteen- and fourteen-year-old kids experimenting with all manners of mood-altering drugs, but they are not drug addicts. They may be at risk or have the potential for the disease of addiction, but they don't have it yet. It is as if the child has high cholesterol but not heart disease. And it is possible to prevent the onset of alcoholism or drug addiction in someone who has the telltale risk factors.

The risks of becoming an alcoholic increase with binge drinking, especially in the formative adolescent years. As biology forms up to 50 percent of one's propensity to develop drug or alcohol addiction, a family history of alcohol or drug misuse is a major red flag.

Other risk factors for teenagers developing drinking problems include low levels of parent supervision or communication, family conflicts, inconsistent or severe parental discipline, problems managing impulses, emotional instability, thrill-seeking behaviors, and perceiving the risk of using alcohol to be low.

Girls whose mothers have drinking problems are at severe risk of alcoholism, as are those who begin drinking before age fourteen. Family relationships, part of the social aspect of contributing factors, indicate that sixteen- to eighteen-year-olds are less prone to excessive drinking if they have a close relationship with their mother.

The treatment appropriate for a binge-drinking teen or a fourteen-year-old who was caught experimenting with cocaine must be entirely different from the treatment given to a middle-aged alcoholic with decades of continual consumption or a thirty-year-old heroin addict with hepatitis C and HIV or to the bipolar twenty-three-year-old who snorts ketamine on the weekend.

The most common reason teenagers end up in rehab is that

they got into trouble at school or home because of their use of alcohol or drugs. Their behavior could range from normal teen experimentation and recklessness to blatantly extreme intoxication and dangerous behavior.

Although drinking does not equal alcoholism and drug use does not equal drug addiction, there is significant pressure to treat the drinking or drugging teen as an alcoholic or addict who must, for his or her own good, be sent off to rehab, even if that treatment is coerced. A current advertisement for a drug and alcohol treatment center in California states, "Even if you have to admit the teen into the facility *against their will*, it will be best for them to be there."

A 1979 U.S. Supreme Court decision gave parents power to commit children who are under age eighteen into a facility without judicial proceedings. This has been a gold mine for private "treatment centers," private mental health facilities, and lawyers specializing in helping parents have their children involuntarily admitted to rehab centers or mental hospitals.

In the past few years, several states have revised their involuntary commitment laws, making it very easy to have loved ones treated for substance misuse, even if they don't want to be treated. According to guidelines in many states, insisting that you don't need treatment is simply proof that you don't realize that you need treatment.

This approach has been hailed by concerned parents as a blessing, because it allows them to get their kids or other family members the help they need. Yet, there is no recognized definition of "the help they need," and many doctors who treat alcoholism and addiction share serious concerns regarding the ethics and wisdom of the state being permitted to institute preventive therapeutic programs against a citizen's will.

Setting aside the ethical issue of coerced admission, there is documentation that drug and alcohol treatment may be equally effective whether admission to the program is voluntary or not. The educational and empowering experience of appropriate treatment can have significant value in helping the teenager consciously choose which behaviors to continue and which to abandon.

If the treatment experience serves only to reinforce an addict/alcoholic identity and continually places the teen in both emotional and social proximity to those with more advanced drug use, the risk of actually becoming an addict or alcoholic in his or her adult years increases.

A teen-only facility also has its challenges. Recent research cautions grouping high-risk teens in peer-group preventive interventions. Such groupings have been shown to produce negative outcomes, as participants reinforce each other's drug use. This must be taken into serious consideration when structuring the interaction of patients at an inpatient treatment center.

The most common drug and alcohol treatment for teens, and everyone else, is a twenty-eight-day program. However, there is no rational or medical reason for twenty-eight days; it is simply the number of days that most insurance companies will cover without objection. When a treatment center advises you that they offer immediate *evaluation*, they don't mean *diagnosis* of the patient's condition. If they meant diagnosis, they would say diagnosis. By *evaluation*, they often mean evaluation of your insurance coverage.

Addiction: False Assumptions

Once in a drug and alcohol treatment center based on the assumption that you are an addict or alcoholic, you are regarded as such, and any protest to the contrary is deemed denial. This approach is most common at 12-step programs or facilities that have a one-size-fits-all concept of treatment.

American psychologist David Rosenhan is known for an eponymous experiment in which he assigned a group of his graduate psychology students to admit themselves into a mental institution, reporting that they were suffering from psychotic symptoms. Once on the psychiatric wards, they behaved in completely normal ways that betrayed absolutely no psychotic symptoms. The medical staff did not realize that these students were normal, diagnosed their behaviors as psychoses, and in fact, refused to let the students leave until they acknowledged and accepted their diagnoses.

Having been sent off to rehab, where they are told that they're "crazy" addicts, a hair's breadth from being failures for the rest of their lives, teenagers return home to discover that everyone else believes the negative labels about them as well. They might as well wear a giant red "A" for "Addict" on their T-shirts.

Post-rehab self-consciousness and depression, accompanied by strong bouts of shame over being such a loser, can cause extreme emotional stress. The post-rehab teen always has one group ready to accept her—those who drink and drug.

"My parents sent me to rehab when I was 13 for issues that could have easily been solved with therapy, family therapy and time," a young woman commented in an online forum. "After I got home from rehab, at age 14, I felt like a huge outcast and was suspended from a school because they found out I went to rehab."

The True First Step to Teen Treatment

Before a teenager is compelled into rehab, the parent or guardian should consult a physician specializing in addiction medicine and engage the teen in full participation with the physician. Consultation and diagnosis by a medical professional is always the best idea. If the teen isn't an alcoholic or an addict, the doctor will say so and will advise the patient regarding whatever medical issues are involved and how to decrease the risks of chronic illness. If the teen is an alcoholic or addict, an addiction medicine specialist is best qualified to recommend the treatment regimen best suited to the individual patient.

Not all teen drinkers will become alcoholics, but all teen drinkers are at risk for a wide variety of health problems and legal sanctions for dangerous behavior. The most comprehensive approach to the reality of teen drug and alcohol use is short-term harm-reduction and commonsense preventive measures to reduce the risks of alcoholism and addiction.

A Family History of Addiction

A wealthy woman had an eighteen-year-old son, Sean, who battled a severe cocaine habit. She had tried to get him into rehab for several years without success. Finally, an intervention was performed, and he was checked into a high-priced facility, where all costs were nonrefundable. Over the weekend, when family members were allowed to visit patients, the mother brought her son a reward for going to rehab—a $25,000 Rolex watch.

You can probably guess what happened. He signed out of the rehab, sold the Rolex, and went on a cocaine binge. This behavior may be immoral, but it is perfectly understandable. Addicts and alcoholics have structural or functional damage to the reward and motivation centers of their brains, located in a part of the brain known as the limbic lobe. When working properly, this reward system causes us to remember and return to pleasurable, life-affirming experiences. When the reward center is damaged, we keep doing things even when the result is pain instead of pleasure.

When I met Sean shortly after his Rolex binge, he was noticeably high. His medical exam confirmed what everyone already knew—he was a cocaine addict but also drank alcohol, popped pills, and smoked marijuana. "I don't discriminate, doc. Whatever I can get my hands on," he said with a grin.

As it turns out, Sean's family had a history of addiction. His maternal aunt died of a heroin overdose. A cousin on his father's side died in an alcohol-related car death; both of his parents were in recovery. I explained to Sean how his uncontrollable drinking and drugging were symptoms of a chronic disease and in his case, one likely with a very strong genetic basis. The fact that he couldn't stop drinking and drugging didn't make him a loser, and it wasn't his fault.

He was stunned and took a minute to absorb this. "Really?

'Cause the last rehab clinic that I went to said it was all my fault and if I really wanted to stop, I would," he said.

I explained that while his disease was not his fault, unfortunately, he was at risk of profound brain damage if he continued drinking and drugging obsessively, because of his relative youth. "You're actually on a rapid pathway to lowering your I.Q., not to mention increasing your risk for need of a liver transplant and shrinking your testicles. If you continue, soon you will be a dumber, sicker, and more impotent version of yourself."

I got his attention. With his parents' consent, I prescribed a regimen of pharmaceutical medications to stop his cravings for drink and drugs. I also arranged for him to begin motivational therapy and got him thinking about a lifestyle modification. We helped him focus on substituting an adrenaline rush through intense exercise (he favored rock climbing) for intoxication through drink and drugs.

Deep down Sean was motivated to quit. He had seen up close the damage substance addiction had caused to his family. Six months after our initial visit, he enrolled in college and is working toward a degree in criminology and forensics science. Yes, he wants to work in criminal justice.

Critical Thinking About Kids and Addiction

Families need to understand the disease of addiction and have realistic expectations of behavior change. This is accomplished when families are well-informed participants in their loved one's treatment.

Critical thinking is also an integral part of evidence-based medical practice. Obviously, we need an increase in critical-thinking abilities, in addition to factual information, to counter the prevalence of harmful ideas regarding addiction, dependence, and treatment.

Booze and the Adolescent Brain

Alcohol and drug abuse causes so much adolescent brain damage that, if we had any sense at all, we would lock up all teenagers until their brains were fully developed in their early twenties. Since that's not going to happen, the next best thing is to inform teens—and adults—of the awful, unvarnished truth.

Adolescence is a unique time in the development of the human brain. Research shows that excessive use of alcohol and drugs results in abnormalities in brain functioning, including structure and volume, white matter quality, and the ability to perform cognitive tasks.

By *abuse,* we don't mean alcohol or drug consumption on the order of adult addiction. As little as one year of heavy drinking, meaning four to five drinks of alcohol a week, can cause the neurodevelopment damage just described. Particularly damaging were bouts of binge drinking where four to five alcoholic drinks are consumed in a short period of time.

Typical adolescent brain development marks a period of accelerated evolution between childhood and adulthood. Complex social, biological, and psychological changes are intertwined, impacting behavior. In short, both biology and environment heighten the adolescent's risk for beginning and abusing alcohol and drugs.

Scientific literature suggests that much of the damage to the brain once done in adolescence cannot be undone. One study showed that even after four weeks of monitored abstinence, youth who had indulged in heavy marijuana use performed worse on performance tests of learning, cognitive flexibility, visual scanning, and working memory than youth who did not smoke marijuana. Similar results have been found with alcohol.

Advances in neuroimaging, like MRI tests, make it easy to identify the parts of the brain affected by alcohol and drug abuse. Let's break it down:

Hippocampus: Research shows that the hippocampus, the part of the brain responsible for memory and spatial navigation, has a measurable decrease in volume among teens who drink and drug heavily, affecting both short-term and long-term memory.

Prefrontal cortex: The frontal lobe is the part of the brain associated with reward, attention, planning, and motivation. As with the hippocampus, heavy teen drinkers and marijuana smokers had smaller frontal lobes than nonusers, resulting in poorer verbal memory. The difference was particularly pronounced among women.

White matter: White matter matters because it regulates the speed of nerve transmission to the brain from elsewhere in the body. Again, teens who are heavy users of alcohol and marijuana have a lower volume of white matter than nonusers, resulting in increased symptoms of depression.

Brain blood flow: Chronic alcoholics have been shown to have reduced blood flow to their brains. Both binge drinking and long-term heavy drinking can lead to strokes, even in people without coronary heart disease. Recent studies show that people who binge drink are about 56 percent more likely than people who never binge drink to suffer an ischemic stroke over ten years. Binge drinkers also are about 39 percent more likely to suffer any type of stroke than people who never binge drink. A recent study examining adolescent women who were heavy drinkers confirmed that their relative youth did not protect them from decreased cerebral blood flow and its potentially damaging effects.

The takeaway here is that current research clearly indicates that heavy alcohol and drug use during adolescence leads to abnormalities in the brain that are not likely to diminish over time.

Chapter 10

Fetal Alcohol Syndrome: Real and Preventable

If there's any underage group that deserves special consideration in any discussion of the disease of addiction, it's the unborn. You may be thinking that this statement is leading to a prolife or prochoice view on the rights of the unborn fetus and the mother. But the point that I'm about to make has nothing to do with partisan politics and everything to do with preventing a devastating condition that it is 100 percent preventable.

In 1968, Christy Ulleland, chief resident at Harborview Medical Center, University of Washington, first discovered the link between prenatal alcohol exposure and adverse outcomes in infants. In January 1968, Ulleland received funding to conduct an eighteen-month study to scientifically assess her clinical observation that infants born to alcoholic women had impaired outcomes. Her conclusion: "Chronic alcoholism can be appropriately added to the list of maternal factors that create an unhealthy intrauterine environment for the developing fetus; the consequences of which may be life long."

Fetal alcohol syndrome (FAS) is the most common preventable cause of mental retardation in the United States, as well as the most preventable cause of birth defects and developmental disabilities.

If you are pregnant or planning to become pregnant, you must absolutely not touch a drop of alcohol. There is no safe amount of alcohol at any time during pregnancy. Not a glass of pinot, a small vodka martini, a glass of hard cider, or a bottle of hand-craft beer. *There is no safe amount of alcohol while you're pregnant.*

It is an established fact, beyond dispute, that even the slightest amount of alcohol, depending on the metabolism of the mother, can cause irreversible birth defects in her child, especially in the first trimester of pregnancy. A baby can emerge from a drinking mother's womb appearing perfectly normal on the outside, but damage to the baby's brain is permanent and irreversible.

There is nothing complex to preventing FAS. All you have to do is not drink alcohol while pregnant. If you can simply refrain from alcohol, you can prevent your child from alcohol-caused mental retardation, physical disabilities, and possible future behavioral problems leading to problems with the law.

Many mothers stop drinking only after they know they are pregnant, but damage to the developing fetus may already have been done. The Surgeon General's recommendation is that a woman refrains from drinking during pregnancy and even earlier if she is planning to become pregnant.

Once again, there is an enormous gap between what people believe and what is actually true. Many people mistakenly believe that mothers of children born with FAS were all heavy drinkers or full-blown alcoholics. This is a false and dangerous belief.

The degree of damage depends on the metabolism and liver functioning of the mother during pregnancy, and no two women are exactly alike. As you don't know details of your metabolism or liver functioning, there is no way to know the severity of damage to your child by having a drink. Drinking a wine cooler while pregnant is not much different from placing a handgun in front of a baby, spinning the cylinder, closing your eyes, pulling the trigger, and hoping to hear *click* while having no idea how many chambers, if any, are empty.

Even brief exposures to small amounts of alcohol may kill brain cells in a developing fetus. A study carried out by John Olney, at the Washington University School of Medicine in St. Louis, showed that just two drinks consumed during pregnancy may be enough to kill some developing brain cells, leading to permanent brain damage.

The Canadian Paediatric Society found that "Fetal alcohol syndrome (FAS) is a common yet under-recognized condition resulting from maternal consumption of alcohol during pregnancy. While preventable, FAS is also disabling. FAS diagnostic and treatment services require a multidisciplinary approach, involving physicians, psychologists, early childhood educators, teachers, social service professionals, family therapists, nurses and community support circles."

All of those diagnostic and treatment services would be

unnecessary if women would simply not drink while pregnant, if they plan on becoming pregnant, or run the possibility of becoming pregnant.

There are really only two reasons why a pregnant woman would drink despite being informed and warned about FAS and the risk of brain damage and mental retardation. The first reason would be that the woman understands the danger but is willing to put her child's brain at risk in exchange for the pleasure she derives from drinking.

The second reason would be that the mother, despite understanding the danger, has the medical illness of alcohol addiction known as alcoholism. The addict cannot stop without professional medical help. If you are pregnant and can't stop drinking, get help immediately.

Devastating Life-Long Brain Damage

Another problem that doctors face in alerting women to the very real danger of FAS is the culture of disbelief resulting from the media-driven "crack baby" scare of the 1980s. The process of medical research that disproved the crack-baby myth is the same process of professional research that has continually proven the truth of FAS and has taught us that fetal alcohol syndrome isn't a single birth defect. It's a cluster of related problems and the most severe of a group of consequences of prenatal alcohol exposure. Collectively, the range of disorders is known as fetal alcohol spectrum disorders (FASDs).

As with the illness of addiction, both the physical and

functional brain damage of FAS can be seen with brain imaging technology. According to a study recently published by a team of researchers at the University of Washington, it is possible to differentiate FASD-diagnosed brains from normal brains with 80 percent accuracy using magnetic resonance imaging of the brain.

The most devastating disability caused by a mother's prenatal use of alcohol is the organic brain damage that impairs an individual's executive brain function—the ability to understand and adapt to the world. A consideration of the following incidents of disease, while more accurate in the generality than the specificity, will give you a sense of perspective.

On any given day in the United States, 10,657 babies are born. Of these, 1 is HIV positive, 2 are born with spina bifida, 3 are born with muscular dystrophy, 10 are born with Down's syndrome, and 120 are born with FAS- or alcohol-related neurodevelopment disorder. It's the number one cause of mental retardation in United States.

The Institute of Medicine's report to Congress on FAS made it clear that the incidence figures were to give a sense of perspective and "to emphasize the magnitude of a problem that has serious implications—for the individual and for society."

Life Problems End Only at Death

Individuals with FASD have problems planning and organizing information in their daily lives, have trouble comprehending the consequences of their behavior, and act on impulse with diminished control. According to expert Kay Kelly, project director of the FAS/FAE Legal Issues Resource Center at the University of Washington, "These individuals typically have an excessive desire to please others, an attitude that may lead them to take (or acquiesce in) actions that are harmful to their own interests."

The social skills of people damaged in the womb by alcohol destine them for a difficult life, despite having an average IQ. "Most individuals with average IQ lead productive and organized lives," says Kelly. "Individuals who have an average IQ but who also have brain damage caused by alcohol in uteri, often struggle unsuccessfully to deal with the usual demands of life."

Easy Prey for Predators

The behavioral disabilities make people with FAS, be they children or adults, easy prey for criminals and perverts. They are more likely to put up with abuse and not complain about it because they don't want to upset the person abusing them. They want to keep people happy and be accepted. Hence they are easily exploited. Some 7 percent of adolescents and adults with FAS or fetal alcohol effects (FAEs) have been physically or sexually abused. Sexual abuse of children with FASD by adults in their own home is a particularly serious problem.

In the court system or in law enforcement, victims or witnesses with FASD can compromise cases because they are eager to please and are very believable. They may think that the "right answer" to a question is the answer the questioner wants to hear. To the FAS person, he or she is not lying, but simply giving the proper answer.

For the millions of individuals who already have FAS, it is too late to protect them from the harm that maternal alcohol caused in their developing brains. But it is still possible to take effective measures to protect them from criminal abuse.

Adults with FAS, if left to fend for themselves, will too often end up living on the streets or, in other circumstances, where they are likely to be particularly vulnerable to crime. The social services that many of these adults need, ranging from supported community living environments to job training, are as important to preventing victimization as they are to preventing poverty.

Studies of FAS in the United States, Canada, and elsewhere portray horrific medical and social consequences for the innocent victims of their mothers' drinking. Children afflicted with full-blown FAS display both physical and mental abnormalities. Those with partial FAS may not have the obvious physical characteristics, but they suffer the same behavioral and psychological problems. These include a low IQ, difficulty in learning from experience, poor judgment, poor cause-and-effect reasoning, and an unawareness of the consequences of behavior. Obviously, these are the very attributes that can lead them to prison.

A child born with FAS will also be an adult with FAS. The condition cannot be cured; it doesn't get better. People born with FAS are very impulsive and do things without thinking about consequences. They are not malicious in their behavior. In fact, they are usually exploited by more talented criminals to do some of the running, or high-risk tasks, and are more likely to get caught.

As many as half the young offenders appearing in court may be there because their mothers drank during pregnancy, says psychologist Josephine Nanson of the Royal Hospital in British Columbia, Canada, who with four of her colleagues conducted a study of 207 cases of FAS over two years. Her assessment could have tremendous implications for how the criminal justice system handles youth in custody.

"The criminal justice system is based on the premise that people understand there are rules, why they have to be obeyed, and if they aren't obeyed then society has the right to come up with any number of options," said Canadian Legal Aid Commission lawyer Kearney Healy, in an interview with the Saskatoon *Star Phoenix* newspaper about Nanson's study. "All of those things are irrelevant to these kids. It's got nothing to do with good or bad—they just don't see it the same way. There are an increasing number of cases reaching the courts because we've been diagnosing this for about 20 years. Those individuals are now in adolescence and adulthood, and at a prime age for when they're going to be involved in the court system."

For every full-blown case of FAS, it is estimated there are four with partial effects.

One of the ironies is that children with FAS often make model prisoners because they do very well in structured environments. "Often people are fooled in the early stages of treatment into thinking somebody is doing really well, not realizing that they're doing really well because all the opportunities for them *not* to do well are taken care of in a structured program," Nanson told the newspaper "This is an illusion. The FAS individual will fall apart emotionally outside that system.

Ignorance Will Send Your Child to Prison

Popular misconceptions about mental illness and mental retardation are partially responsible for railroading FAS sufferers through the criminal justice system. From arrest to the determination of competency to stand trial and beyond, a person's mental health affects every stage of passage through the criminal justice system.

If you doubt that assertion, simply ask yourself whether or not mentally ill people act weird, peculiar, or suspicious. Does the behavior of people with mental problems attract attention? Of course it does, and that includes attracting police attention, even if a crime hasn't been committed.

Untrained to recognize and handle mental illness, be it caused by exposure to alcohol in the womb or any other factor, arresting officers and other staff inappropriately assume the arrestee understands such things as their Miranda rights. Children and adults with FAS are more likely to give false confessions simply to please the police.

A Public Health Issue

Even the brief review presented here should prove adequate to make my case: FAS is a devastating problem with a dreadful impact on millions of lives. All the pain, suffering, punitive measures, imprisonment, and fortunes spent on researching effective ways to treat FAS would all vanish in a generation if women simply didn't drink alcohol before or during pregnancy. Not one drop. Not one beer. No loving mother would trade her child's future for a six-pack, a wine cooler, or a bottle of single malt scotch.

Defining the Problem of Fetal Alcohol Disorders

For purposes of distinction, the term FAS is commonly used for the condition in which there are distinctive facial abnormalities that may be discerned by a trained medical expert. These facial features include small eyes, an exceptionally thin upper lip, a short, upturned nose, and a smooth skin surface between the nose and upper lip.

Doctors have used a number of terms to describe some of the signs of fetal alcohol syndrome and the spectrum of disorders caused when a pregnant woman consumes alcohol, such as fetal alcohol spectrum disorders (FASD), fetal alcohol syndrome (FAS), fetal alcohol effects (FAEs), partial fetal alcohol syndrome (pFAS), alcohol-related neurodevelopmental disorders (ARNDs), static encephalopathy alcohol exposed (SEAE), and alcohol-related birth defects (ARBDs). ARND refers to mental and behavioral impairments; ARBD refers to the physical defects that occur from fetal alcohol exposure. Most of these characteristics are not characterized by the telltale facial features and require a higher level of testing and evaluation.

Signs of fetal alcohol syndrome may include the following:

- Heart defects
- Deformities of joints, limbs, and fingers
- Slow physical growth before and after birth
- Vision difficulties or hearing problems

- Small head circumference and brain size (microcephaly)
- Poor coordination
- Sleep problems
- Mental retardation and delayed development
- Learning disorders
- A short attention span, hyperactivity, and poor impulse control
- Extreme nervousness and anxiety

The facial features seen with fetal alcohol syndrome may also occur in healthy children without FAS. Distinguishing normal facial features from those of FAS requires expertise.

Opiate Addiction during Pregnancy

Although less widespread than FAS, opiate drug use among pregnant women is a rapidly growing problem.

The number of women abusing opiates increased 500 percent between 2000 and 2009, according to the National Institute on Drug Abuse. It's estimated that 75 percent of all heroin addicts who are pregnant never receive any prenatal care.

Health risks for a baby born of a mother abusing opiates include learning disabilities, behavioral problems, and mental or physical developmental delays.

A pregnant woman addicted to opiates should go through withdrawal for her own health and that of her unborn child, and she should do it between the fourteenth and thirty-second weeks to minimize the effect on the fetus. (If she doesn't detox before birth, her newborn baby is likely to be born addicted and will have to go through a withdrawal process, which can take weeks.) The pregnant mother's detox must be done under the supervision of a physician who is trained and board-certified in addiction medicine. One other option is during pregnancy to stay on Subutex or methadone maintenance because in some individuals detox is more painful and even dangerous to the mother and fetus. Again, the objective is to do no harm; which option is better depends on the patient.

Overcoming the Culture of Disbelief

These are strange days for practitioners of addiction medicine like myself. We find ourselves living in a kind of twilight between the past and future. We're surrounded by hordes of zombie rehab clinics that offer antiquated remedies for what should be the medical treatment of addiction. Even our own medical brethren too often hear only the siren call of the 12 steps and ignore their Hippocratic Oath to do no harm by discharging their addicted patients into the hands of amateurs.

In short, we live in a culture of disbelief, where medical science about addiction is cast aside.

Dramatic? Perhaps. But I really do believe we're in the midst of an epic struggle for the treatment of addiction. I have been fighting the battle now for fifteen years. I was among the first doctors to begin treating patients with a substance addiction with controlled and scientifically verified medications like Suboxone.

And it's been twenty-five years since the advent of magnetic resonance imaging proved what doctors of addiction medicine had always suspected: The brain of the alcohol and drug addict is structurally different from that of a nonaddict's.

Decades now into the struggle to make evidence-based medicine the default treatment for substance addiction, the other side still seems to be winning. Incredibly, 90 percent of all rehab clinics and treatment centers for alcohol and drug addiction offer no evidence-based medicine. The largely unregulated, $34 billion rehab industry can make more profit by refusing to recognize the science of addiction treatment. The worst of the lot have simply co-opted and commodified the simple 12-step philosophy—meant always to have been a free program as much about sanctuary and camaraderie as about treatment—into a program offered as a cure and run by drug counselors with no medical training. The more sophisticated ones offer psychological counseling staffed by degreed therapists, but most still ignore the irrefutable research that medications are an essential part of a comprehensive treatment. I know from talking to their former patients that many facilities in Los Angeles where I live won't even allow their doctors to talk about medications.

More troubling, we're drowning in new waves of substance addiction. Suburban youth are now the new poster children for the flood of cheap and powerful heroin flooding the streets. Late-middle-aged to senior adults—traditionally the last group you would think of as drug addicts—are hooked on powerful prescription painkillers with the rate of OD deaths for those ages fifty-five to sixty-four soaring 700 percent between 1993 and 2012. (In 2012, Medicare spent zero on powerful tranquilizers such as Xanax and

Valium; one year later, under pressure from the pharmaceutical companies to include their products in Medicare authorized medication, it was spending $377 million on 40 million prescriptions for this class of drugs.)

Hundreds of thousands of veterans are being treated for substance addictions of all kinds. The nation's energy boom has been accompanied by a methamphetamine epidemic among gas and oil workers. One study, reported in the *Wall Street Journal*, found nearly 25 percent of federally mandated energy workers testing positive for amphetamine in 2011, up from 17 percent just two years earlier.

As for alcohol, it now has the dubious distinction of being the third leading preventable cause of death in the United States, surpassed only by smoking and obesity and responsible for nearly 88,000 deaths in 2014. That's more than deaths from firearms, drug abuse, and sexually transmitted diseases combined (alcohol-related deaths surpassed those from car accidents in 2011 and never looked back). Heavy drinking is up more than 17 percent since 2005, with women registering the biggest increases. That is particularly saddening but not surprising since the prevalence of fetal alcohol syndrome has also risen over the last decade from approximately 3 cases per 1,000 to as high as 7 cases per 1,000 (the more broadly defined fetal alcohol spectrum disorder is as high as 50 cases per 1,000).

A complicit judiciary continues to condition people's freedom on attendance to 12-step programs rather than bona fide, evidence-based treatment centers. Quite literally, people are dying every day because of ill-informed, sometimes religiously biased and often politically cynical elected judges who kowtow to constituents who expect addicts to be demonized as criminals rather than treated as patients.

The death rate from drug overdoses more than doubled from 1999 to 2013. The nation spends nearly $468 billion annually on addiction but only 2¢ goes for prevention or long-term treatment (the rest is squandered on jails, courts, and emergency care at hospitals).

Yet, maddeningly, after all these years the public at large remains confused about addiction and its treatment. Many people do not believe that addiction is a physical disease, but that is only because they don't understand the meaning of disease and the current definition of addiction. Surveys show that the majority of Americans understand that addiction has a biological component—that it's a disease like diabetes, asthma, or bipolar disorder—yet they can't let go of the past. They cling to the notion that addicts could really stop if they wanted to and that willpower and moral fiber are the answers to substance addiction.

The destined-to-fail war on drugs and its sister campaigns DARE and Just Say No are twentieth-century relics, dismissed by anyone under thirty years old with the same derision my generation had for *Reefer Madness*. Yet, politicians continue to pay homage to these failed public health policies.

Hope on the Horizon

Still, I am hopeful about the changing landscape of addiction treatment. There is a new class of warriors who are fighting for science and medicine and the treatment of addiction as the chronic disease that it is. I know this because I teach med students and residents every semester at the University of Southern California Keck School of Medicine. The school is at the forefront of informing their soon-to-be doctors about the disease of addiction and the evidence-based treatments available. Indeed, every med student at the school, no matter what his or her intended specialty, must take the curriculum that I, along with my staff, created.

We also now have a history of how evidence-based treatment can, and has, worked. Thousands of patients who likely would have been jailed or succumbed to the ravages of substance addiction are now living normal lives. Medications such as Suboxone have been developed to stop the cravings that characterize substance addiction without the danger of a new dependency.

The concept of substance addiction as a chronic disease that must be treated over a lifetime, as is the case with every other chronic disease, has gained a toehold in popular culture. The failure of local and state authorities to use evidence-based treatment has been chronicled recently in investigative news articles in the *Huffington Post*, *Slate*, *The Atlantic* magazine, and the *New York Times*, with the cumulative effect of casting doubt on the invulnerability of the 12-step monolith.

Documentary films such as *The Business of Recovery* directed by Adam Finberg and *Prescription Thugs* by Chris Bell, Josh Alexander, and Craig Young question the motives behind both the rehab industry and big pharma.

Most heartening, the treatment of addiction as a medical condition is becoming institutionalized. The federal Affordable

Care Act (Obamacare), for the first time in national healthcare policy, mandated what health benefits insurance plans must cover, and substance addiction treatment is included. What's more, it bars insurers from denying coverage due to preexisting conditions—including substance abuse.

But perhaps the most important changes emanating from President Obama's landmark healthcare initiative is the expansion of the so-called parity rules. *Parity* means that insurance plans must cover mental health and substance abuse treatment at the same level as regular medical care. Once and for all, after a century of needless criminalization, the Affordable Care Act codifies in federal law that substance abuse is a medical issue—not the result of moral turpitude and not a problem meant for the criminal justice system.

Finally, under the Affordable Care Act, insurance will pay for evidence-based treatment. Already, some of the most famous and egregious proponents of the 12-step abstinence-only model for treatment are quickly changing their tune. Hazelden, the first center to, in effect, co-opt Bill Wilson's AA philosophy and charge money for it, has now incorporated naltrexone into its treatment model. Big health insurers like Cigna and United Healthcare are following the new law and simply refusing to pay for inpatient treatment claims from centers that do not use evidence-based medicine. Soon, AA will return to what its founder always meant it to be—a free service that might help heavy drinkers and even some alcoholics, rather than being enshrined as the foundation for a nationwide for-profit industry that exploits the fears and suffering of addicts and their families.

The irrationality of drug criminalization is being embraced by a younger generation of Americans. States like Colorado and Washington have decriminalized marijuana use, thus opening it to regulation and taxation (just like alcohol). Similarly, voters in California recently passed Proposition 47 that revises the calculus of drug courts. The new law changed several felonies, including drug possession, into misdemeanors, thus expanding the opportunities for potentially hundreds to receive addiction treatment whose crimes previously were deemed too serious.

Next Steps

So, where do we go from here? First, if you're reading this book because you or someone you care about is an addict, be informed! Choose a treatment center wisely. Do not be swayed by marketing campaigns that gloss over a rehab clinic's failure to provide appropriate medical care. Look for evidence-based treatment not only in the detoxification phase of treatment but also in management and maintenance. Avoid centers that promise only a 12-step model, a one-size-fits-all treatment program, and especially a cure for alcoholism or drug addiction.

As a society, we need to catch up with the rest of the Western world and incorporate commonsense healthcare reform, beyond those offered by the Affordable Care Act, including the following:

1. Require all medical schools to offer a mandatory curriculum on evidence-based addiction treatment. Remember that substance addiction is the third leading cause of

preventable deaths in the United States. It's shameful that only a handful of medical schools offer training to their students, much less require it.

2. Use taxes on the legal sale of marijuana and alcohol for a public education program about the facts concerning the chronic disease that we call alcoholism and drug addiction.

3. Develop standardized terms to facilitate treatment. Too often both the public and doctors interchange terms at random, causing confusion. Not all people who drink or take drugs or who drink heavily or take lots of drugs are addicts. Most of those who consume alcohol and drugs will simply stop or moderate that behavior to a safe level. The term *addict* must be reserved for those who have the chronic, largely genetically based brain disease, characterized by a damaged reward system and an uncontrollable, obsessive craving for a substance.

4. Regulate the alcohol and drug rehab industry. New mandates under the Affordable Care Act will go a long way, but a comprehensive federal law should be passed to require treatment centers to be under the supervision of a medical doctor with a certification in addiction medicine and staffed by trained and licensed medical professionals. The days when your only qualification for being an addiction counselor is that you used to be an addict, or still are, must end.

A Universal Problem

Addiction, as with other chronic clinical illnesses, doesn't consider your race, religion, or political affiliation. It doesn't matter if someone is Christian, Jewish, Muslim, Buddhist, Hindu, or atheist. This disease afflicts people from all walks of life, rich and poor, doctors, successful businessmen, clergy, and elected heads of state. The more people know about the disease of addiction, the less stigmatized individuals who suffer from it will be, and more will get the help they need (keep in mind that 90 percent of those who suffer from the disease are not being treated at all).

Every physician and clinical association worldwide recognizes that substance addiction is a clinical illness that is both preventable and treatable. It is to this mission of prevention and treatment that I have dedicated my life and career, and I invite you to join me as an ambassador of the truth about addiction.

BIBLIOGRAPHY

Aalto, M., Pekuri, P., & Seppa, K. (2003). "Obstacles to carrying out brief intervention for heavy drinkers in primary health care: A focus group study." *Drug and Alcohol Review* 22 (2): 169–73.

Abbott, P. J., Quinn, D., & Knox, L. (1995). "Ambulatory medical detoxification for alcohol." *American Journal of Drug & Alcohol Abuse* 21 (4): 549–63.

Abraham, A. J., & Roman, P. M. (2010). "Early adoption of injectable naltrexone for alcohol-use disorders: Findings in the private-treatment sector." *Journal of Studies on Alcohol and Drugs* 71 (3): 460–66.

Abraham, A. J., Knudsen, H. K., & Roman, P. M. (2011). "A longitudinal examination of alcohol pharmacotherapy adoption in substance use disorder treatment programs: Patterns of sustainability and discontinuation." *Journal of Studies on Alcohol and Drugs* 72 (4): 669–77.

Adams, J. B., Heath, A. J., Young, S. E., Hewitt, J. K., Corley, R. P., & Stallings, M. C. (2003). "Relationships between personality and preferred substance and motivations for use among adolescent substance abusers." *American Journal of Drug and Alcohol Abuse* 29 (3): 691–712.

Agrawal, A., & Lynskey, M. T. (2008). "Are there genetic influences on addiction: Evidence from family, adoption and twin studies." *Addiction* 103 (7): 1069–81.

Alcoholics Anonymous World Services. (1972). *A Brief Guide to Alcoholics Anonymous.*

Alexander, J. A., Nahra, T. A., Lemak, C. H., Pollack, H., & Campbell, C. I. (2008). "Tailored treatment in the outpatient substance abuse treatment sector: 1995–2005." *Journal of Substance Abuse Treatment* 34 (3): 282–92.

Amato, L., Davoli, M., Perucci, C. A., Ferri, M., Faggiano, F., & Mattick, R. P. (2005). "An overview of systematic reviews of the effectiveness of opiate maintenance therapies: Available evidence to inform clinical practice and research." *Journal of Substance Abuse* 28 (4): 321–29.

American Board of Addiction Medicine Foundation. (2009). *The Need for Addiction Medicine Physicians and for Addiction Medicine Residency Training Programs: A Report of the American Board of Addiction Medicine Foundation.* Chevy Chase, MD.

American Medical Association. (2011). H-95.976. "Drug abuse in the United States: The next generation." Available at ssl3.ama-assn.org.

American Medical Association, Council on Scientific Affairs. (1979). *Guidelines for Alcoholism Diagnosis: Treatment and Referral.* Chicago.

American Psychiatric Association. (2008). "Substance use disorders: Physician performance measurement set: PCPI approved." Available at www.ama-assn.org.

American Society of Addiction Medicine. (2011). "Definition of addiction: Frequently asked questions." Available at www.asam.org.

Anderson, A. L., Reid, M. S., Li, S. H., et al. (2009). "Modafinil for the treatment of cocaine dependence." *Drug and Alcohol Dependence* 104 (1–2): 133–39.

Anonymous. (2012, February 22). "A rewired brain: Many now see addiction as a chronic brain disease that requires new approaches to treatment." *Wall Street Journal.* Available at http://online.wsj.com/ad/cigna/cigna_article.htm.

Anthony, E. K., Taylor, S. A., & Raffo, Z. (2011). "Early intervention for substance abuse among youth and young adults with mental health conditions: An exploration of community mental health practices." *Administration and Policy in Mental Health* 38 (3): 131–41.

Anton, R. F., Moak, D. H., Latham, P., et al. (2005). "Naltrexone combined with either cognitive behavioral or motivational enhancement therapy for alcohol dependence." *Journal of Clinical Psychopharmacology* 25 (4): 349–57.

Anton, R. F., & Swift, R. M. (2003). "Current pharmacotherapies of alcoholism: A U.S. perspective." *American Journal on Addictions* 12 (1): S53–S68.

Appel, P. W., Ellison, A. A., Jansky, H. K., & Oldak, R. (2004). "Barriers to enrollment in drug abuse treatment and suggestions for reducing them: Opinions of drug injecting street outreach clients and other system stakeholders." *American Journal of Drug and Alcohol Abuse* 30 (1): 129–53.

Arias, A. J., & Kranzler, H. R. (2008). "Treatment of co-occurring alcohol and other drug use disorders." *Alcohol Research and Health* 31 (2): 155–67.

Atkinson, R. M., Ganzini, L., & Bernstein, M. J. (1992). "Alcohol and substance-use disorders in the elderly." In J. E. Birren, R. B. Sloane, & G. D. Cohen, eds., *Handbook of Mental Health and Aging* (pp. 516–55). New York: Academic Press.

Azrin, N. H., Sisson, W., Myers, R., & Godley, M. (1982). "Alcoholism treatment by disulfiram and community reinforcement therapy." *Journal of Behavior Therapy and Experimental Psychiatry* 13 (2): 105–12.

Babor, T. F., & Hall, W. (2007). "Editorial: Standardizing terminology in addiction science: To achieve the impossible dream." *Addiction* 102 (7): 1015–18.

Babor, T. F., & Kadden, R. M. (2005). "Screening and interventions for alcohol and drug problems in medical settings: What works?" *Journal of Trauma* 59 (Suppl. 3): S80–S87.

Barker, M. J., Greenwood, K. M., Jackson, M., & Crowe, S. F. (2004). "Cognitive effects of long-term benzodiazepine use. A meta-analysis." *CNS Drugs* 18 (1): 37–48.

Barnett, P. G., Zaric, G. S., & Brandeau, M. L. (2001). "The cost-effectiveness of buprenorphine maintenance therapy for opiate addiction in the United States." *Addiction* 96 (9): 1267–278.

Bava, S., Frank, L. R., McQueeny, T., Schweinsburg, B. C., Schweinsburg, A. D., & Tapert, S. F. (2009). "Altered white matter microstructure in adolescent substance users." *Psychiatry Research* 173 (3): 228–37.

Bazelon Center for Mental Health Law. (2010). "Medicaid reforms in the Patient Protection and Affordable Care Act and the Health Care and Education Reconciliation Act." Available at www.bazelon.org.

Bellack, A. S., Bennett, M. E., Gearon, J. S., Brown, C. H., & Yang, Y. (2006). "A randomized clinical trial of a new behavioral treatment for drug abuse in people with severe and persistent mental illness." *Archives of General Psychiatry* 63 (4): 426–32.

Biery, J. R., Williford, J. H., Jr., & McMullen, E. A. (1991). "Alcohol craving in rehabilitation: Assessment of nutrition therapy." *Journal of the American Dietetic Association* 91 (4): 463–66.

Bina, R., Yum, J., Hall, D., Sowbel, L., et al. (2008). "Substance abuse training and perceived knowledge: Predictors of perceived preparedness to work in substance abuse." *Journal of Social Work Education* 44 (3): 7–20.

Bishop, E. S. (1919). "Narcotic drug addiction: A public health problem." *American Journal of Public Health* 9 (7): 481–88.

Block, M. A. (1956). "Medical treatment of alcoholism." *JAMA* 162 (18): 1610–619.

Boden, M. T., Kimerling, R., Jacobs-Lentz, J., et al. (2011). "Seeking safety treatment for male veterans with a substance use disorder and post-traumatic stress disorder symptomology." *Addiction* 107 (3): 578–86.

Boden, M. T., & Moos, R. (2009). "Dually diagnosed patients' responses to substance use disorder treatment." *Journal of Substance Abuse Treatment* 37 (4): 335–45.

Bodenheimer, T., Wagner, E. H., & Grumbach, K. (2002). "Improving primary care for patients with chronic illness: The chronic care model, Part 2." *JAMA* 288 (15): 1909–914.

Bollerud, K. (1990). "A model for the treatment of trauma-related syndromes among chemically dependent inpatient women." *Journal of Substance Abuse Treatment* 7 (2): 83–87.

Bonnie, R. J., & O'Connell, M. E. (2004). *Reducing underage drinking: A collective responsibility.* Washington, D.C.: National Academies Press.

Boothby, L. A., & Doering, P. L. (2007). "Buprenorphine for the treatment of opioid dependence." *American Journal of Health-System Pharmacy* 64 (3): 266–72.

Bowen, O. R., & Sammons, J. H. (1988). "The alcohol-abusing patient: A challenge to the profession." *JAMA* 260 (15): 2267–270.

Brady, J. P., Posner, M., Lang, C., & Rosati, M. J. (1994). *Risk and reality: The implications of prenatal exposure to alcohol and other drugs.* Rockville, MD: U.S. Department of Health and Human Services and the U. S. Department of Education, Educational Development Center.

Brown, B. S., & Flynn, P. M. (2002). "The federal role in drug abuse technology transfer: A history and perspective." *Journal of Substance Abuse Treatment* 22 (4): 245–57.

Brown, J. D., Vartivarian, S., & Alderks, C. E. (2011). "Child care in outpatient substance abuse treatment facilities for women: Findings from the 2008 National Survey of Substance Abuse Treatment Services." *Journal of Behavioral Health Services & Research* 38 (4): 478–87.

Brown, R. L., Leonard, T., Saunders, L. A., & Papasouliotis, O. (1998). "The prevalence and detection of substance use disorders among inpatients ages 18 to 49: An opportunity for prevention." *Preventive Medicine* 27 (1): 101–10.

Buck, J. A. (2011). "The looming expansion and transformation of public substance abuse treatment under the affordable care act." *Health Affairs* 30 (8): 1402–410.

Buddy, T. (2010). "Naltrexone—Treatment for alcoholism and addiction: Blocks effects of opioids, reduces alcohol craving." Available at alcoholism.about.com.

Buddy, T. (2007). "New vaccines help stop drug addiction?" Available at alcoholism.about.com.

Burge, S. K., & Schneider, F. D. (1999). "Alcohol-related problems: Recognition and intervention." *American Family Physician* 59 (2): 361–70, 372.

Burke, B. L., Arkowitz, H., & Menchola, M. (2003). "The efficacy of motivational interviewing: A meta-analysis of controlled clinical trials." *Journal of Consulting and Clinical Psychology* 71 (5): 843–61.

Burrow-Sanchez, J., Call, M. E., Adolphson, S. L., & Hawken, L. S. (2009). "School psychologists' perceived competence and training needs for student substance abuse." *Journal of School Health.*

Burrow-Sanchez, J. J., & Lopez, A. L. (2009). "Identifying substance abuse issues in high schools: A national survey of high school counselors." *Journal of Counseling and Development* 87 (1): 72–79.

Burton, L. M. (1992). "Black grandparents rearing children of drug-addicted parents: Stressors, outcomes, and social service needs." *Gerontologist* 32 (6): 744–51.

Busto, U., Sellers, E. M., Naranjo, C. A., Cappell, H., Sanchez-Craig, M., & Sykora, K. (1986). "Withdrawal reaction after long-term therapeutic use of benzodiazepines." *New England Journal of Medicine* 315 (14): 854–59.

Calhoun, P. S., Elter, J. R., Jones, E. R. Jr., Kudler, H., & Straits-Troster, K. (2008). "Hazardous alcohol use and receipt of risk-reduction counseling among U.S. veterans of the wars in Iraq and Afghanistan." *Journal of Clinical Psychiatry* 69 (11): 1686–693.

Califano, J. A. (2007). *High society: How substance abuse ravages America and what to do about it.* New York: Public Affairs.

California Board of Behavioral Sciences. (2012). "Continuing education (CE) provider application." Available at www.bbs.ca.gov.

Callahan, D. (1999). "Remembering the goals of medicine." *Journal of Evaluation in Clinical Practice* 5 (2): 103–106.

Carey, K. B. (2008, December 22). "Drug rehabilitation or revolving door?" *New York Times*, p. 1D.

Carey, K. B., Bradizza, C. M., Stasiewicz, P. R., & Maisto, S. A. (1999). "The case for enhanced addictions training in graduate programs." *Behavior Therapist* 22 (2): 27–31.

Carroll, K. M. (1996). "Relapse prevention as a psychosocial treatment: A review of controlled clinical trials." *Experimental and Clinical Psychopharmacology* 4 (1): 46–54.

Carroll, K. M., Ball, S. A., Nich, C., et al. (2001). "Targeting behavioral therapies to enhance naltrexone treatment of opioid dependence: Efficacy of contingency management and significant other involvement." *Archives of General Psychiatry* 58 (8): 755–61.

Carroll, K. M., Fenton, L., Ball, R. (2004). "Efficacy of disulfiram and cognitive behavior therapy in cocaine-dependent outpatients: A randomized placebo-controlled trial." *Archives of General Psychiatry* 61 (3): 264–72.

Carroll, K. M., Rounsaville, B. J., Nich, C., Gordon, L., & Gawin, F. (1995). "Integrating psychotherapy and pharmacotherapy for cocaine dependence: Results from a randomized clinical trial." *NIDA Research Monograph* 150: 19–35.

CASAColumbia (2012). "Addiction medicine: Closing the gap between science and practice. Results from a 5-year study." Available at http://www.casacolumbia.org/addiction-research/reports/addiction-medicine.

Cassel, E. J. (1982). "The nature of suffering and the goals of medicine." *New England Journal of Medicine* 306 (11): 639–45.

Catholic University of America. (2010). "Summary of federal laws.

The Controlled Substances Act of 1970 (Title II of the Comprehensive Drug Abuse Prevention and Control Act of 1970)." Available at counsel.cua.edu.

Center for Substance Abuse Treatment. (2011). "About buprenorphine therapy." Available at buprenorphine.samhsa.gov.

Center for Substance Abuse Treatment. (2005). "Acamprosate: A new medication for alcohol use disorders (DHHS Pub. No. (SMA) 05-4114)." *Substance Abuse Treatment Advisory* 4 (1).

Center for Substance Abuse Treatment. (2012). "Buprenorphine information center." Available at buprenorphine.samhsa.gov.

Center for Substance Abuse Treatment. (2004). *Clinical guidelines for the use of buprenorphine in the treatment of opioid addiction. Treatment improvement protocol (TIP) Series 40* (DHHS Pub. No. (SMA) 04-3939). Rockville, MD: U.S. Department of Health and Human Services, Substance Abuse and Mental Health Services Administration, Center for Substance Abuse Treatment.

Center for Substance Abuse Treatment. (1997). *A guide to substance abuse services for primary care clinicians. Treatment improvement protocol (TIP) Series 24* (DHHS Pub. No. (SMA) 97-3139). Rockville, MD: U.S. Department of Health and Human Services, Substance Abuse and Mental Health Services Administration, Center for Substance Abuse Treatment.

Center for Substance Abuse Treatment. (2000). *Improving substance abuse treatment: The national treatment plan initiative: Changing the conversation* (DHHS Pub No. (SMA) 00-3480, NCADI Pub No. -BKD 383). Rockville, MD: U.S. Department of Health and Human Services, Substance Abuse and Mental Health Services Administration, Center for Substance Abuse Treatment.

Center for Substance Abuse Treatment. (2009). *Incorporating alcohol pharmacotherapies into medical practice. Treatment Improvement Protocol (TIP) Series 49.* (DHHS Pub. No. (SMA) 09-4380). Rockville, MD: U.S. Department of Health and Human Services, Substance Abuse and Mental Health Services Administration.

Center for Substance Abuse Treatment. (2006). "Prescription medications: Misuse, abuse, dependence, and addiction." *Substance Abuse Treatment Advisory* 5 (2): 1–4.

Center for Substance Abuse Treatment. (1994). *Screening and assessment for alcohol and other drug abuse among adults in the criminal justice system. Treatment improvement protocol (TIP) Series 7* (DHHS Pub. No. (SMA) 94-2076). Rockville, MD: U.S. Department of Health and Human Services, Substance Abuse and Mental Health Services Administration, Center for Substance Abuse Treatment.

Center for Substance Abuse Treatment. (1998). *Substance abuse among older adults. Treatment improvement protocol (TIP) Series 26* (DHHS Pub. No. (SMA) 98-3179). Rockville, MD: U.S. Department of Health and Human Services, Substance Abuse and Mental Health Services Administration, Center for Substance Abuse Treatment.

Center for Substance Abuse Treatment. (2005). *Substance abuse treatment for persons with co-occurring disorders. Treatment improvement protocol (TIP) Series 42* (DHHS Pub. No. (SMA) 05-3992). Rockville, MD: U.S. Department of Health and Human Services, Substance Abuse and Mental Health Services Administration, Center for Substance Abuse Treatment.

Centers for Disease Control and Prevention, National Center for Injury Prevention and Control. (2011). "Prescription painkiller overdoses in the U.S." Available at www.cdc.gov.

Chambers, R. A., Taylor, J. R., & Potenza, M. N. (2003). "Developmental neurocircuitry of motivation in adolescence: A critical period of addiction vulnerability." *American Journal of Psychiatry* 160(6): 1041–1052.

Cherkis, Jason. (2015, January 28) "Dying to be free—There's a treatment for heroin addiction that actually works. Why aren't we using it?" *Huffington Post.* Available at http://projects.huffing tonpost.com/dying-to-be-free-heroin-treatment.

Clark, R. E., Samnaliev, M., Baxter, J. D., & Leung, G. Y. (2011). "The evidence doesn't justify steps by state Medicaid programs to restrict opioid addiction treatment with buprenorphine." *Health Affairs* 30 (8): 1425–433.

Comer, S. D., Sullivan, M. A., Yu, E., et al. (2006). "Injectable, sustained-release naltrexone for the treatment of opioid dependence: A randomized, placebo-controlled trial." *Archives of General Psychiatry* 63 (2): 210–18.

Courtwright, D. T. (2001). *Dark Paradise: A History of Opiate Addiction in America.* Cambridge: Harvard University Press.

Crews, F. T., & Boettiger, C. A. (2009). "Impulsivity, frontal lobes and risk for addiction." *Pharmacology Biochemistry and Behavior* 93 (3): 237–47.

Crews, F., He, J., & Hodge, C. (2007). "Adolescent cortical development: A critical period of vulnerability for addiction." *Pharmacology Biochemistry and Behavior* 86 (2): 189–99.

Culberson, J. W., & Ziska, M. (2008). "Prescription drug misuse/abuse in the elderly." *Geriatrics* 63 (9): 22–31.

Cunningham, J. A., Sobell, L. C., Sobell, M. B., Agrawal, S., & Toneatto, T. (1993). "Barriers to treatment: Why alcohol and drug abusers delay or never seek treatment." *Addictive Behaviors* 18 (3): 347–53.

Cunningham, R. M., Harrison, S. R., McCay, M. P., et al. (2010). "National survey of emergency department alcohol screening and intervention practices." *Annals of Emergency Medicine* 55 (6): 556–62.

Curtis, J. R., Geller, G., Stokes, E. J., Levine, D. M., & Moore, R. D. (1989). "Characteristics, diagnosis, and treatment of alcoholism in elderly patients." *Journal of the American Geriatrics Society* 37 (4): 310–16.

Dackis, C. A., Lynch, K. G., Yu, E., et al. (2003). "Modafinil and cocaine: A double-blind, placebo-controlled drug interaction study." *Drug and Alcohol Dependence* 70 (1): 29–37.

Dackis, C., & O'Brien, C. P. (2005). "Neurobiology of addiction: Treatment and public policy ramifications." *Nature Neuroscience* 8 (11): 1431–436.

Dahl, R. E. (2004). "Adolescent brain development: A period of vulnerabilities and opportunities. Keynote address." *Annals of the New York Academy of Sciences* 1021: 1–22.

Denizet-Lewis, B. (2006, June 25). "An anti-addiction pill?" Available at www.nytimes.com.

Devenyi, P., Mitwalli, A., & Graham, W. (1982). "Clonidine therapy for narcotic withdrawal." *Canadian Medical Association Journal* 127 (10): 1009–1011.

DeWit, D. J., Adlaf, E. M., Offord, D. R., & Ogborne, A. C. (2000). "Age at first alcohol use: A risk factor for the development of alcohol disorders." *American Journal of Psychiatry* 157 (5): 745–50.

Dhalla, I. A. (2011). "Facing up to the prescription opioid crisis." *British Journal of Medicine* 343 (d5142).

Dowling, G. J., Weiss, S., & Condon, T. P. (2008). "Drugs of abuse and the aging brain." *Neuropsychopharmacology* 33 (2): 209–18.

Drake, R. E., Mercer-McFadden, C., Mueser, K. T., McHugo, G. J., & Bond, G. R. (1998). "Review of integrated mental health and substance abuse treatment for patients with dual disorders."

Drug Policy Alliance. (2009). "Healing a broken system: Veterans battling addiction and incarceration." Available at www.phoe nixhouse.org.

Druss, B. G., & Mauer, B. J. (2012). "Health care reform and care at the behavioral health–primary care interface." *Psychiatric Services* 61 (11): 1087–1092.

Dufour, M. C., Archer, L., & Gordis, E. (1992). "Alcohol and the elderly." *Clinics in Geriatric Medicine* 8 (1): 127–41.

Dupont, R. L., McLellan, A. T., Carr, G., Gendel, M., & Skipper, G. E. (2009). "How are addicted physicians treated? A national survey of physician health programs." *Journal of Substance Abuse Treatment* 37 (1): 1–7.

Elisnon, Zusha. (2015, March 16). "Aging baby boomers bring drug habits into middle age." *Wall Street Journal.* Available at http:// www.wsj.com/articles/aging-baby-boomers-bring-drug-habits -into-middle-age-1426469057.

Epstein, J., Barker, P., Vorburger, M., & Murtha, C. (2004). *Serious mental illness and its co-occurrence with substance use disorders, 2002* (DHHS Publication No. SMA 04-3905, Analytic Series A-24). Rockville, MD: U.S. Department of Health and Human Services, Substance Abuse and Mental Health Services Administration, Office of Applied Studies.

Ersche, K. D., Jones, P. S., Williams, G. B., Turton, A. J., Robbins, T. W., & Bullmore, E. T. (2012). "Abnormal brain structure implicated in stimulant drug addiction." *Science* 335 (6068): 601–604.

Finlayson, R. E., Hurt, R. D., Davis, L. J., & Morse, R. M. (1988). "Alcoholism in elderly persons: A study of the psychiatric and psychosocial features of 216 inpatients." *Mayo Clinic Proceedings* 63 (8): 761–68.

Finney, J. W., Wilbourne, P. L., & Moos, R. H. (2007). "Psychosocial treatments for substance use disorders." In P. E. Nathan & J. M. Gorman, eds., *A Guide to Treatments That Work* (pp. 179–202). New York: Oxford University Press.

Fiorentine, R. (1999). "After drug treatment: Are 12-step programs effective in maintaining abstinence?" *American Journal of Drug and Alcohol Abuse* 25 (1): 93–116.

Fournier, M. E., & Levy, S. (2006). "Recent trends in adolescent substance use, primary care screening, and updates in treatment options." *Current Opinions in Pediatrics* 18 (4): 352–58.

Galanter, M., Dermatis, H., Glickman, L., et al. (2004). "Network therapy: Decreased secondary opioid use during buprenorphine maintenance." *Journal of Substance Abuse Treatment* 26: 313–18.

Ganju, V. (2006). "Mental health quality and accountability: The role of evidence-based practices and performance measures." *Administration and Policy in Mental Health* 33 (6): 659–65.

Glaser, Gabrielle. (April 2015). "The irrationality of Alcoholics Anonymous." *The Atlantic*. Available at http://www.theatlantic .com/magazine/archive/2015/04/the-irrationality-of-alcoholics -anonymous/386255.

Haber, P. (2012). "Pharmacotherapies for alcohol dependence." In E. Proude, O. Loptko, N. Lintzeris, & P. Haber, eds., *Guidelines for the Treatment of Alcohol Problems: A Review of Evidence* (pp. 169–72). Sydney, Australia: University of Sydney.

Han, B., Gfroerer, J. C., & Colliver, J. D. (2010). "Associations between duration of illicit drug use and health conditions: Results from the 2005–2007 National Surveys on Drug Use and Health." *Annals of Epidemiology* 20 (4): 289–97.

Han, B., Gfroerer, J. C., Colliver, J. D., & Penne, M. A. (2009). "Substance use disorder among older adults in the United States in 2020." *Addiction* 104 (1): 88–96.

Hankin, J. R. (2002). "Fetal alcohol syndrome prevention research." *Alcohol Research and Health* 26 (1): 58–65.

Holder, H. D. (1998). "Cost benefits of substance abuse treatment: An overview of results from alcohol and drug abuse." *Journal of Mental Health Policy & Economics* 1 (1): 23–29.

Holloway, H. C., Hales, R. E., & Watanabe, H. K. (1984). "Recognition and treatment of acute alcohol withdrawal syndromes." *Psychiatric Clinics of North America* 7 (4): 729–43.

Hommer, D. W., Bjork, J. M., & Gilman, J. M. (2011). "Imaging brain response to reward in addictive disorders." *Annals of the New York Academy of Sciences* 1216: 50–61.

Hoof-Haines, K. V. (2012). "Dual diagnosis: The status of treating co-occurring disorders in the U.S." Available at www.drug free.org.

Jerrell, J. M., & Ridgely, M. S. (1995). "Comparative effectiveness of three approaches to serving people with severe mental illness and substance abuse disorders." *Journal of Nervous and Mental Disease* 183 (9): 566–76.

Johnson, B. A. (2005). "Recent advances in the development of treatments for alcohol and cocaine dependence: Focus on topiramate and other modulators of GABA or glutamate function." *CNS Drugs* 19 (10): 873–96.

Johnson, B. A. (2008). "Update on neuropharmacological treatments for alcoholism: Scientific basis and clinical findings." *Biochemical Pharmacology* 75 (1): 34–56.

Johnson, B. A., & Ait-Daoud, N. (1999). "Medications to treat alcoholism." *Alcohol Research and Health* 23 (2): 99–106.

Johnson, R. E., Chutuape, M. A., Strain, E. C., Walsh, S. L., Stitzer, M. L., & Bigelow, G. E. (2000). "A comparison of levomethadyl acetate, buprenorphine, and methadone for opioid dependence." *New England Journal of Medicine* 343 (18): 1290–297.

Jones, H. E. (2004). "Practical considerations for the clinical use of buprenorphine." *Science and Practice Perspectives* 2 (2): 4–20.

Kalivas, P. W., & Vokow, N. D. (2005). "The neural basis of addiction: A pathology of motivation and choice." *American Journal of Psychiatry* 162 (8): 1403–413.

Kampman, K. M. (2008). "The search for medications to treat stimulant dependence." *Addiction Science and Clinical Practice* 4 (2): 28–35.

Kampman, K. M., Pettinati, H., Lynch, K. G., et al. (2004). "A pilot trial of topiramate for the treatment of cocaine dependence." *Drug and Alcohol Dependence* 75 (3): 233–40.

Karila, L., Reynaud, M., Aubin, H. J., et al. (2011). "Pharmacological treatments for cocaine dependence: Is there something new?" *Current Pharmaceutical Designs* 17 (14): 1359–368.

Karila, L., Weinstein, A., Aubin, H. J., Benyamina, A., Reynaud, M., & Batki, S. L. (2010). "Pharmacological approaches to methamphetamine dependence: A focused review." *British Journal of Clinical Pharmacology* 69 (6): 578–92.

Kaskutas, L. A. (2009). "Alcoholics Anonymous effectiveness: Faith meets science." *Journal of Addictive Disorders* 28 (2): 145–57.

Kelley, A. E., & Berridge, K. C. (2002). "The neuroscience of natural rewards: Relevance to addictive drugs." *Journal of Neuroscience* 22 (9): 3306–311.

Kelly, J. F., Magill, M., & Stout, R. L. (2009). "How do people recover from alcohol dependence? A systematic review of the research on mechanisms of behavior change in Alcoholics Anonymous." *Addiction Research and Theory* 17 (3): 236–59.

Kelly, J. F., & Yeterian, J. D. (2011). "The role of mutual-help groups in extending the framework of treatment." Available at pubs .niaaa.nih.gov.

Keyes, K. M., Hatzenbuehler, M. L., McLaughlin, K. A., et al. (2010). "Stigma and treatment for alcohol disorders in the United States." *American Journal of Epidemiology* 172 (12): 1364–372.

Khantzian, E. J. (1985). "The self-medication hypothesis of addictive disorders: Focus on heroin and cocaine dependence." *American Journal of Psychiatry* 142 (11): 1259–264.

Kjome, K. L., & Moeller, F. G. (2011). "Long-acting injectable naltrexone for the management of patients with opioid dependence." *Substance Abuse: Research and Treatment* 5: 1–9.

Kleber, H. D., Weiss, R. D., Anton, R. F., et al. (2006). "Part A: Treatment of patients with substance use disorders, second edition." American Psychiatric Association. *American Journal of Psychiatry* 163 (Suppl. 8): 5–82.

Knudsen, H. K., Abraham, A. J., Johnson, J. A., & Roman, P. M. (2009). "Buprenorphine adoption in the National Drug Abuse Treatment Clinical Trials Network." *Journal of Substance Abuse Treatment.*

Knudsen, H. K., Abraham, A. J., & Oser, C. B. (2011). "Barriers to the implementation of medication-assisted treatment for substance use disorders: The importance of funding policies and medical infrastructure." *Evaluation and Program Planning* 34 (4): 375–81.

Kosten, T. R., & O'Connor, P. G. (2003). "Management of drug and alcohol withdrawal." *New England Journal of Medicine* 348 (18): 1786–795.

Krishnan-Sarin, S., Krystal, J. H., Shi, J., Pittman, B., & O'Malley, S. S. (2007). "Family history of alcoholism influences naltrexone-induced reduction in alcohol drinking." *Biological Psychiatry* 62 (6): 694–97.

Leshner, A. I. (1997). "Addiction is a brain disease, and it matters." *Science* 278 (5335): 45–47.

———. (1999). "Science is revolutionizing our view of addiction—and what to do about it."

Lindborg, Kristina. (2014, March 28). "Why heroin is spreading in America's suburbs." *Christian Science Monitor*. Available at http://www.csmonitor.com/USA/Society/2014/0323/Why -heroin-is-spreading-in-America-s-suburbs-video.

Ling, W., Charuvastra, C., Collins, J. F., et al. (1998). "Buprenorphine maintenance treatment of opiate dependence: A multicenter, randomized clinical trial." *Addiction* 93 (4): 475–86.

Mangrum, L. F., Spence, R. T., & Lopez, M. (2006). "Integrated versus parallel treatment of co-occurring psychiatric and substance use disorders." *Journal of Substance Abuse Treatment* 30 (1): 79–84.

Miller, W. R., Sorensen, J. L., Selzer, J. A., & Brigham, G. S. (2006). "Disseminating evidence-based practices in substance abuse treatment: A review with suggestions." *Journal of Substance Abuse.*

Millery, M., Kleinman, B. P., Polissar, N. L., Millman, R. B., & Scimeca, M. (2002). "Detoxification as a gateway to long-term treatment: Assessing two interventions." *Journal of Substance Abuse Treatment* 23 (3): 183–90.

Milliken, C. S., Auchterlonie, J. L., & Hoge, C. W. (2007). "Longitudinal assessment of mental health problems among active and reserve component soldiers returning from the Iraq war." *JAMA* 298 (18): 2141–148.

Mroziewicz, M., & Tyndale, R. F. (2010). "Pharmacogenetics: A tool for identifying genetic factors in drug dependence and response to treatment." *Addiction Science & Clinical Practice* 5 (2): 17–29.

Munro, Dan. (2015, April 27). "Inside the $35 billion addiction treatment industry." *Forbes.* Available at http://www.forbes.com/sites/danmunro/2015/04/27/inside-the-35-billion-addiction-treatment-industry.

Narconon International. (2011). History of marijuana. Available at www.narconon.org.

National Center on Addiction and Substance Abuse. (2012). CASA-Columbia report. *Addiction Medicine: Closing the Gap between Science and Practice. Results from a 5-year study.* Available at http://www.casacolumbia.org/addiction-research/reports/addiction-medicine.

National Institute on Drug Abuse. (2005). "Drug abuse and addiction: One of America's most challenging public health problems." Available at www.nida.nih.gov.

National Institute on Drug Abuse. (2011). "Preventing and recognizing prescription drug abuse." Available at www.nida.nih.gov.

National Institute on Drug Abuse. (2012). "Research report series: Heroin abuse and addiction: What are the treatments for heroin addiction?" Available at www.drugabuse.gov.

O'Brien, C. P. & McKay, J. (2007). "Psychopharmacological treatments for substance use disorders." In P. E. Nathan & J. M. Gorman, eds., *A Guide to Treatments That Work* (3rd ed., pp. 145–177). New York: Oxford University Press.

O'Connor, P. G. (2005). "Methods of detoxification and their role in treating patients with opioid dependence." *JAMA* 294 (8): 961–63.

O'Connor, P. G., Carroll, K. M., Shi, Ju. M., Schottenfeld, R. S., Kosten, T. R., & Rounsaville, B. J. (1997). "Three methods of opioid detoxification in a primary care setting: A randomized trial." *Annals of Internal Medicine* 127 (7): 526–30.

O'Connor, P. G., & Fiellin, D. A. (2000). "Pharmacologic treatment of heroin-dependent patients." *Annals of Internal Medicine* 133 (1): 40–54.

O'Connor, P. G., Nyquist, J. G., & McLellan, T. (2011). "Integrating addiction medicine into graduate medical education in primary care: The time has come." *Annals of Internal Medicine* 154 (1): 56–59.

O'Connor, P. J., & Youngstedt, S. D. (1995). "Influence of exercise on human sleep." *Exercise and Sport Sciences Reviews* 23 (1): 105–34.

O'Farrell, T. J., & Fals-Stewart, W. (2003). "Alcohol abuse." *Journal of Marital and Family Therapy* 29 (1): 121–46.

Patterson, T. L., & Jeste, D. V. (1999). "The potential impact of the baby-boom generation on substance abuse among elderly persons." *Psychiatric Services* 50(9): 1184–188.

Pescosolido, B. A., Martin, J. K., Long, J. S., Medina, T. R., Phelan, J. C., & Link, B. G. (2010). "A disease like any other"? A decade of change in public reactions to schizophrenia, depression, and alcohol dependence." *American Journal of Psychiatry* 167 (11): 1321–330.

Petrakis, I. L., Leslie, D., & Rosenheck, R. (2003). "Use of naltrexone in the treatment of alcoholism nationally in the Department of Veterans Affairs." *Alcoholism: Clinical and Experimental Research* 27 (11): 1780–784.

Petrakis, I. L., Rosenheck, R., & Desai, R. (2011). "Substance use comorbidity among veterans with posttraumatic stress disorder and other psychiatric illness." *American Journal on Addictions* 20 (3): 185–89.

Rieckmann, T. R., Kovas, A. E., Fussell, H. E., & Stettler, N. M. (2009). "Implementation of evidence-based practices for treatment of alcohol and drug disorders: The role of the state authority." *Journal of Behavioral Health Services & Research* 36 (4): 407–19.

Roan, S. (2008). "The 30-day myth." *Los Angeles Times.* Available at articles.latimes.com.

Robert Wood Johnson Foundation. (2001). *Substance Abuse: The Nation's Number One Health Problem: Key Indicators for Policy Update.* Princeton, NJ.

SAMHSA's National Registry of Evidence-based Programs and Practices. (2007). "Motivational enhancement therapy (MET)." Available at nrepp.samhsa.gov.

SAMHSA's National Registry of Evidence-based Programs and Practices. (2008). "Multidimensional family therapy (MDFT)." Available at nrepp.samhsa.gov.

SAMHSA's National Registry of Evidence-based Programs and Practices. (2007). "National Registry of Evidence-Based Programs and Practices (NREPP)." Available at nrepp.samhsa.gov.

Scheinholtz, M. K. (2011). "Implementation of evidence-based practices: SAMHSA's older adults targeted capacity expansion grant program." *Journal of the American Society on Aging* 34 (1): 26–35.

Schramm-Sapyta, N. L., Walker, Q. D., Caster, J. M., Levin, E. D., & Kuhn, C. M. (2009). "Are adolescents more vulnerable to drug addiction than adults? Evidence from animal models." *Psychopharmacology* 206 (1): 1–21.

Seal, K. H., Cohen, G., Waldrop, A., Cohen, B. E., Maguen, S., & Ren, L.

(2011). "Substance use disorders in Iraq and Afghanistan veterans in VA healthcare, 2001–2010: Implications for screening, diagnosis and treatment." *Drug and Alcohol Dependence* 116 (1–3): 93–101.

Shen, X., Orson, F. M., & Kosten, T. R. (2011). "Anti-addiction vaccines." *F1000. Medicine Report* 3: 20.

Shorter, D., & Kosten, T. R. (2011). "Vaccines in the treatment of substance abuse." *FOCUS: Journal of Lifelong Learning in Psychiatry* 9 (1): 25–29.

Spohr, H. L., Willms, J., & Steinhausen, H. C. (1993). "Prenatal alcohol exposure and long-term developmental consequences." *Lancet* 341 (8850): 907–10.

Squeglia, L. M., Jacobus, J., & Tapert, S. F. (2009). "The influence of substance use on adolescent brain development." *Clinical Electroencephalography and Neuroscience* 40 (1): 31–38.

Squeglia, L. M., Spadoni, A. D., Infante, M. A., Myers, M. G., & Tapert, S. F. (2009). "Initiating moderate to heavy alcohol use predicts changes in neuropsychological functioning for adolescent girls and boys." *Psychology of Addictive Behaviors* 23 (4): 715–22.

Substance Abuse and Mental Health Services Administration. (2012). "Co-occurring disorders in veterans and military service members." Available at www.samhsa.gov.

Thomas, C. P., Reif, S., Haq, S., Wallack, S. S., Hoyt, A., & Ritter, G. A. (2008). "Use of buprenorphine for addiction treatment: Perspectives of addiction specialists and general psychiatrists."

Timko, C., Moos, R. H., Finney, J. W., & Lesar, M. D. (2000). "Long-term outcomes of alcohol use disorders: Comparing untreated individuals with those in Alcoholics Anonymous and formal treatment." *Journal of Studies on Alcohol* 61 (4): 529–40.

Tsuang, M. T., Bar, J. L., Harley, R. M., & Lyons, M. J. (2001). "The Harvard Twin Study of Substance Abuse: What we have learned." *Harvard Review of Psychiatry* 9 (6): 267–79.

Tsuang, M. T., Lyons, M. J., Harley, R. M., et al. (1999). "Genetic and environmental influences on transitions in drug use." *Behavior Genetics* 29 (6): 473–79.

U.S. Department of Justice, National Drug Intelligence Center. (2010). "Impact of drugs on society." Available at www.justice.gov.

U.S. Department of Veteran Affairs, National Center for PTSD. (2011). "PTSD and problems with alcohol use." Available at www.ptsd.va.gov.

U.S. House of Representatives, Office of the Legislative Counsel. (2010). *Compilation of Patient Protection and Affordable Care Act.* 111th Cong., 2nd Sess. Print 111-111. Available at housedocs.house.gov.

University of Washington, Alcohol and Drug Abuse Institute. (2006). "Evidence-based practices for treating substance use disorders: Matrix of interventions." Available at adai.washington.edu.

van den Bree, M. B., Johnson, E. O., Neale, M. C., & Pickens, R. W. (1998). "Genetic and environmental influences on drug use and abuse/dependence in male and female twins." *Drug and Alcohol Dependency* 52 (3), 231–41.

Van Hoof-Haines, K. (2012). "Dual diagnosis: The status of treating co-occurring disorders in the U.S." Available at www.drugfree.org.

Volkow, N. D. (2007). *Drugs, Brains, and Behavior: The Science of*

Addiction [rev. August 2010] (NIH Pub. No. 10-5605). Rockville, MD: U.S. Department of Health and Human Services, National Institute on Drug Abuse.

Volkow, N. D., & Skolnick, P. (2012). "New medications for substance use disorders: Challenges and opportunities." *Neuropsychopharmacology* 37 (1): 290–92.

Watkins, K., Pincus, H. A., Tanielian, T. L., & Lloyd, J. (2003). "Using the chronic care model to improve treatment of alcohol use disorders in primary care settings." *Journal of Studies on Alcohol*, 64 (2), 209–18.

White, W., & Kurtz, E. (2005). *The Varieties of Recovery Experience: A Primer for Addiction Treatment Professionals and Recovery Advocates.* Chicago: Great Lakes Addiction Technology Transfer Center.

Wilk, J. E., Bliese, P. D., Kim, P. Y., Thomas, J. L., McGurk, D., & Hoge, C. W. (2010). "Relationship of combat experiences to alcohol misuse among U.S. soldiers returning from the Iraq war." *Drug and Alcohol Dependence* 108 (1–2): 115–21.

Willenbring, M. L. (2008). "New research is redefining alcohol disorders: Does the treatment field have the courage to change?" *Addiction Professional* 6 (5): 12–19.

World Health Organization. (2011). "Management of substance abuse. Lexicon of alcohol and drug terms published by the World Health Organization." Available at www.who.int.

Yoast, R. A., Wilford, B. B., & Hayashi, S. W. (2008). "Encouraging physicians to screen for and intervene in substance use disorders: Obstacles and strategies for change." *Journal of Addictive Diseases* 27 (3): 77–97.

Yuferov, V., Levran, O., Proudnikov, D., Nielsen, D. A., & Kreek, M. J. (2010). "Search for genetic markers and functional variants involved in the development of opiate and cocaine addiction and treatment. *Annals of the New York Academy of Sciences* 1187: 184–207.

Zook, C. J., & Moore, F. D. (1980). "High-cost users of medical care." *New England Journal of Medicine* 302 (18): 996–1002.

ACKNOWLEDGMENTS

A book of this scope requires assistance from many.

First, I would like to give special thanks to the team that facilitated its publication, including Greg Ptacek for captaining the book from proposal to final manuscript; my literary agent Harvey Klinger for navigating the project through the ever-changing shoals of today's publishing world; and publisher John Duff for providing the book safe harbor at Penguin Random House.

I also to wish to thank my colleagues at University of Southern California Keck School of Medicine, who have allowed me to create and teach an addiction medicine curriculum that I hope will serve as a model for medical school nationwide. I thank, too, my students for constantly challenging convention and questioning the status quo.

Also deserving praise is the staff at my clinic and our residential facility Inspire Malibu. Their professionalism, expertise, and dedication are hallmarks of our evidence-based treatment program.

Finally, I wish to sincerely thank the patients who allowed me to share their stories here within these pages. To borrow a timeless inscription from ancient Egypt, may they *ankh wedja seneb*: "Live long, be healthy, and prosper."

INDEX

Agency for Healthcare Research and
Quality, 43
alcohol, 34, 51, 138
  bars and nightclubs and, 179–80
  binge drinking and, 72, 164, 176,
    183, 190
  brain and, 18, 59–61
  danger of, 6
  deaths from, ix–x, 6, 33, 36, 59,
    70–71, 207
  dependence on, 20, 60–61
  detoxification from, 124–26
  as different from other drugs,
    30–33
  driving and, 21, 60, 176, 177,
    179–80
  economic cost of, x
  genetics and, 60, 61
  Joanne's experience with, 47–49,
    50, 63
  legal age for drinking, 177–78
  legality and social acceptability of,
    6, 30, 36, 59, 70–71
  length of average addiction to, 176
  marijuana and, 81, 85
  mixing other drugs with, 71
  physical damage from, 59,
    71–72, 74
  pregnancy and, see pregnancy
  Prohibition and, 6, 114
  psychiatric problems and, 73–74
  tolerance to, 60
  withdrawal from, 17–19
alcoholics, 157–58
  anxiety and depression in, 164
  Freud on, 32–33
  rock bottom and, 43–44
  suicide and, 70, 74
Alcoholics Anonymous (AA), 7, 8–10,
  20–21, 24, 28–29, 44–45, 92, 95,
  130, 145, 151, 172, 210
  films and, 15
  Hoffman and, 5
  medications and, 13, 160–61
  problems with, 12–13, 21
  rock bottom and, 43–44

sponsors in, 13
structure and philosophy of, 9,
  12, 210
see also 12-step programs
*Alcoholics Anonymous: The Story of
  How Many Thousands of Men and
  Women Have Recovered from
  Alcoholism* (Big Book), 9–10
alcoholism:
  first use of term, 31
  medications for treatment of, 98,
    115–16
alcohol withdrawal delirium, 124–26
Alertec, 117, 128
Alexander, Josh, 209
Alzheimer's disease, 77, 93
American Academy of Pain
  Medicine, 64
American Board of Addiction
  Medicine, 131, 132, 152
American Medical Association
  (AMA), xi, 3, 131, 138
American Pain Society, 64
American Psychiatric Association,
  3, 138
American Society for Reproductive
  Medicine, 82
American Society of Addiction
  Medicine (ASAM), 64, 66–67,
  96, 120, 140–41
  Patient Placement Criteria of, 141
amphetamines, 77, 78
analgesics, 20, 34, 37
  see also opiates and opioids
anger, 106–11
Antabuse (disulfiram), 116,
  144–45, 170
anxiety, 164
anxiolytic drugs, 20, 34
  see also benzodiazepines
arthritis, 93, 172
assessment for treatment, 95–96
asthma, 1, 14, 23, 30, 31, 43, 49, 51,
  93, 95, 133, 208
Ativan, 125
Atlantic, 41, 209

ABOUT THE AUTHOR

Akikur Mohammad, M.D., is a specialist in addiction medicine and an award-winning academic who has practiced psychiatry, addiction medicine, and general medicine since 1998, when he opened his private practice in Los Angeles. He is board-certified in addiction medicine by the American Board of Addiction Medicine and in psychiatry by the American Board of Psychiatry and Neurology. Dr. Mohammad is Adjunct Clinical Professor at LAC/USC Medical Center, where he is active in teaching medical students and residents in addiction medicine and psychiatry.

He has been honored many times for his dedication to providing superior care and support to his patients and students. He received the Outstanding Teaching Award from USC in 2003, Outstanding Teaching Award from Residents in 2012, and Outstanding Service Award in 2006 for his work as the Associate Director at LAC/USC Medical Center Psychiatric Emergency Services.

Patient's Choice Award has honored him with the Top Psychiatrists of America Award several times since 2005. In 2011, Who's Who in America named Dr. Mohammad the Top Addiction Professional of the Year. In recognition of his thorough knowledge of addiction and psychiatric medicine, Dr. Mohammad has been the guest speaker at numerous regional and national conferences.

He has also appeared on various radio and television programs, including those on ABC, A&E, and MTV.

He founded and serves as the medical director for Inspire Malibu in Los Angeles, a science and evidence-based drug and alcohol treatment facility that focuses on dual-diagnosis and treating patients with addiction and co-occurring disorders. He established the center in 2010 to create an environment where his practice of evidence-based, scientifically advanced addiction medicine could be fully realized.